The peripartum cow

PRACTICAL NOTES

Manuel Fernández Sánchez
Manuel Liz López
Matilde Hernández Solís

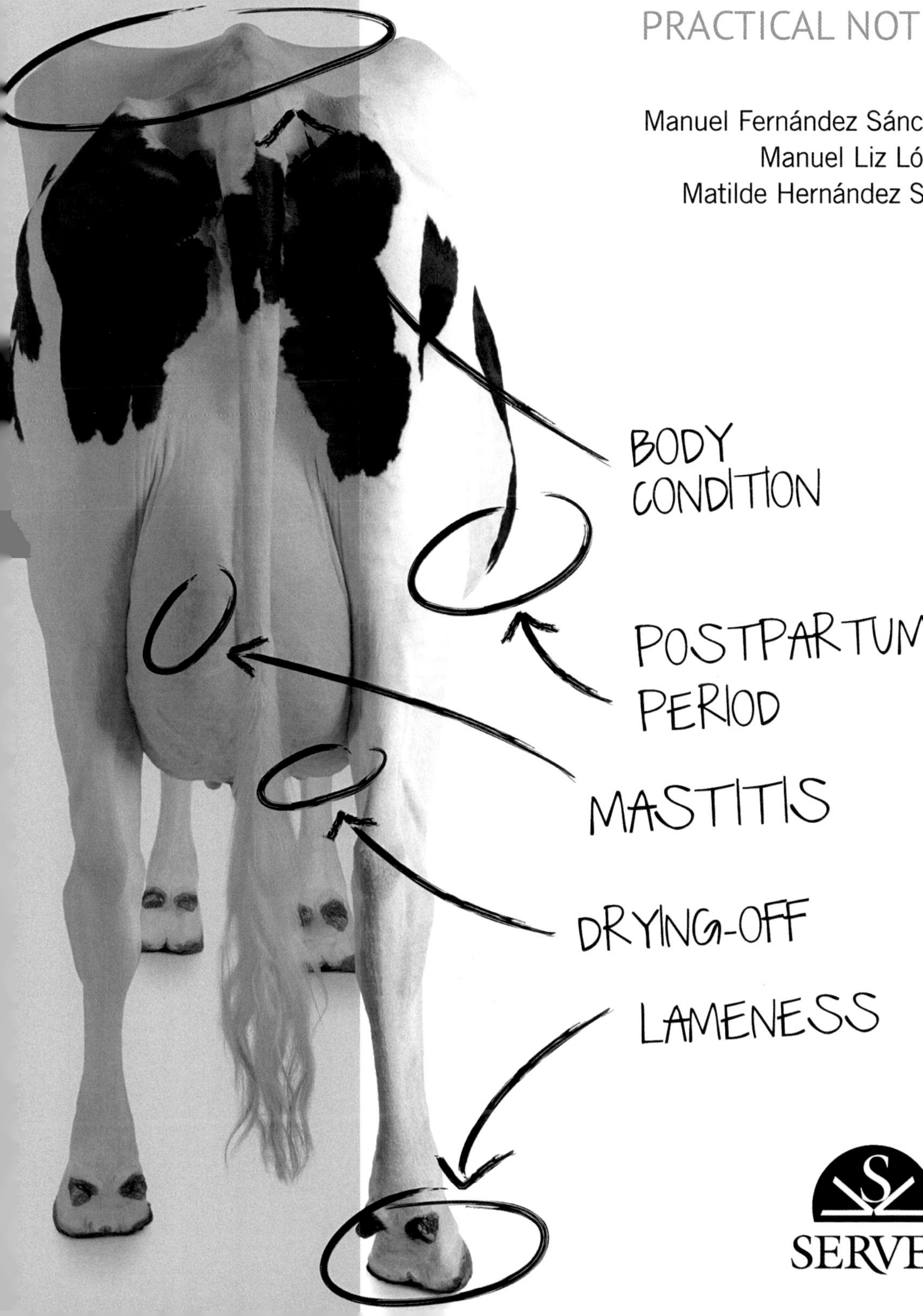

SERVET

Warning:
Veterinary science is constantly evolving, as are pharmacology and the other sciences. Inevitably, it is therefore the responsibility of the veterinary clinician to determine and verify the dosage, the method of administration, the duration of treatment and any possible contraindications to the treatments given to each individual patient, based on his or her professional experience. Neither the publisher nor the author can be held liable for any damage or harm caused to people, animals or properties resulting from the correct or incorrect application of the information contained in this book.

This book has been published originally in Spanish under the title:
El periparto de la vaca. Apuntes prácticos

ISBN spanish edition: 978-84-941014-6-5

For this English edition:

Plaza Antonio Beltrán Martínez nº 1, planta 8 - letra I
(Centro empresarial El Trovador)
50002 Zaragoza - Spain

Translation: Owen Howard

Design and layout:
Servet editorial - Grupo Asís Biomedia, S.L.
www.grupoasis.com
info@grupoasis.com

ISBN: 978-84-942449-6-4
D.L.: Z 786-2014

Printed in Spain

Dedicated to Francisco Hernández Macarro.

Mati and Manolo especially thank their colleagues at Servepo for their patience and understanding during the writing of this book.

Thanks also to Segundo, Susana, Sito, Patricia and Noé.

Preface

In this book, we share our views on the most important part of the production cycle of the cow: the peripartum period. A multidisciplinary approach is the only way to cover all fronts for a successful peripartum management.

The state of the legs, udder health, the type of food and housing provided, and other sufficiently stressful factors can trigger a metabolic cascade of one disease after another.

The solution to these problems proposed here is the formation of a strong support network between veterinary specialists and farmers.

The authors

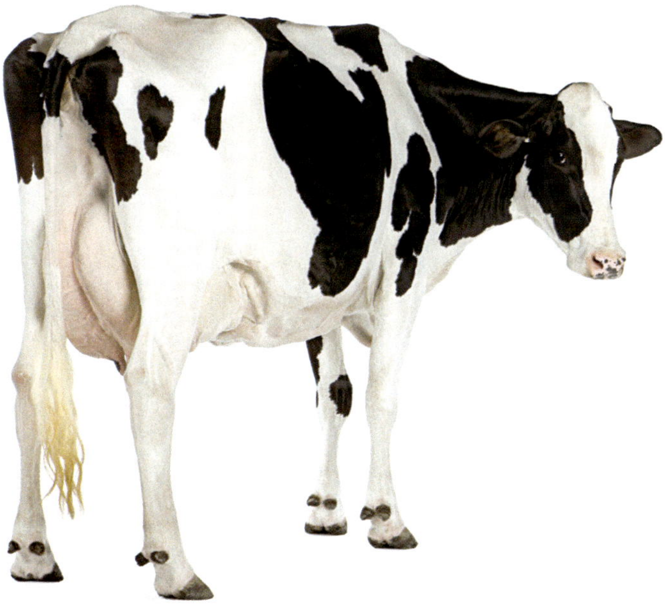

Authors

Manuel Fernández Sánchez

Bachelor of Veterinary Science from the University of Zaragoza. His career, spanning 20 years, has centred on the world of ruminants, from his work in practices in Bristol, Belgium and Scotland to his current role as Ruminant Technical Manager at Evialis Galicia.

He has worked with ANGRA (National Association of Farmers of Rasa Aragonesa sheep) developing breeding and reproduction programmes in meat sheep, and in Asturias overseeing the reproduction and milk quality of dairy cattle.

This professional experience in diverse business areas, clinical practice and in dairy cattle breeding have provided him with a broad vision of the needs of the veterinary surgeons, particularly when it comes to solving problems of a reproductive nature. In this book, he draws upon his experience as a clinician dealing with real problems in the field.

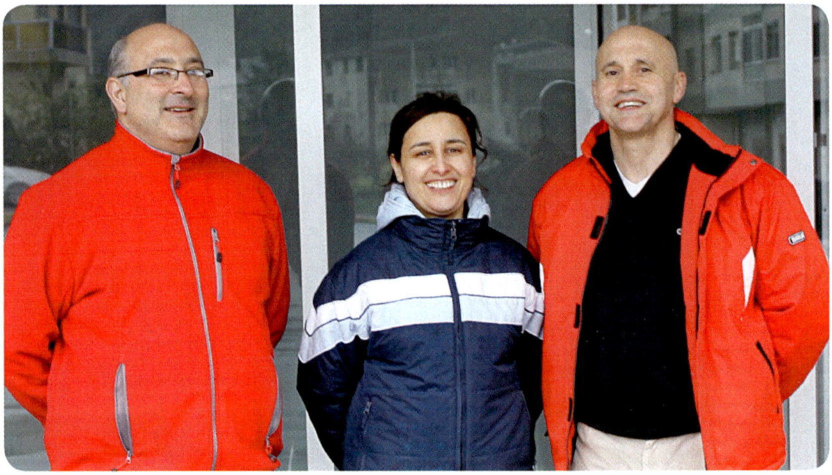

Manuel Liz López

Bachelor of Veterinary Science from the University of León, 1988, the year he began his career as a clinical veterinary surgeon working with dairy and beef cattle in the province of Lugo. He is a founding member of Pontenova Veterinary Services. In his daily work, he alternates between roles as a clinical veterinary surgeon and reproduction specialist. Throughout his career he has participated in numerous training courses and seminars in pathology, surgery, ultrasound and cattle farm management.

Matilde Hernández Solís

Bachelor of Veterinary Science from the University of León, 1989. Since then she has worked as a large animal clinician, and has specialised in milk quality since 2003, when she launched a programme to improve the quality of milk in 70 cattle farms in the province of Lugo. She has been a partner at Pontenova Veterinary Services since 2008. She is also a researcher on the R&D project "Influence of milking equipment on milk production and health status of dairy cattle herds in Galicia: economic impacts on farms (2007-2010)" for Pontenova Veterinary Services.

Table of contents

7 CASE STUDIES

1 Introduction

From an economic viewpoint, the lifespan of a cow can be divided into productive periods (lactation) and non-productive periods (before the first calving, rearing, and the dry period) (Fig. 1).

The term non-productive, however, is perhaps a thankless way to describe the phase during which crucial preparations for lactation are made. Moreover, rearing is a crucial phase from the economic point of view, as it is important that the female calf develops into a well-sized milk-producing cow.

Once the rearing stage is completed, each lactation presents a new challenge. Cows must be dried off and adapted after each lactation. This requires a well-coordinated multidisciplinary team to ensure that the necessary adjustments are performed both rapidly and effectively. The milk quality consultant recommends the necessary treatments and the dry-off protocol, while the nutritionist advises the best approach to ration adaptation. The podiatrist is responsible for treating the hooves, while the clinician plays a key role in both the prevention (e.g. scheduled vaccinations, antiparasitic treatments, etc.) and treatment of diseases, providing the necessary support so that the cow can best recover from the trauma of calving and avoid or overcome potential postpartum clinical problems.

In general, farmers tend to attach more importance to immediate issues (producing lots of milk) than to less pressing but nonetheless crucial concerns (e.g. the unproductive periods that facilitate milk production), perhaps unaware that one extra litre per day at peak lactation can produce an extra 200 litres over the entire lactation period, or that fertility can be improved if peak lactation is reached earlier.

A book like this one is necessary to go further into the most important aspect of lactation, the preparatory phase, which encompasses drying-off, calving, and the peripartum period. These are crucial stages in the life cycle of every dairy cow.

Figure 1. Productive and non-productive periods in the cow.

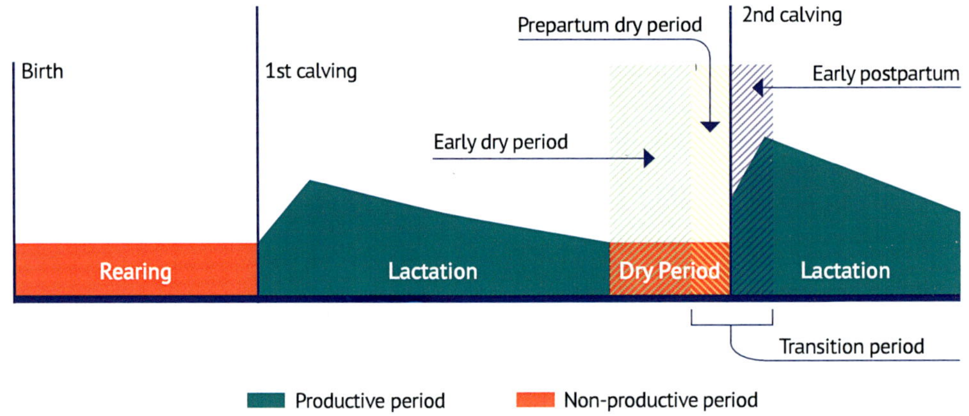

If all professional personnel (not only the farmer) involved in the preparation of the cow achieve a better understanding of this process, the goal of this book will have been accomplished.

> Preparation of the cow for lactation requires special attention during the dry period, calving, and the peripartum period.

The stages of the peripartum period

Diseases that occur during the peripartum period are not independent events. It is very difficult to describe a specific disease process in the peripartum cow without referring to its interaction with other processes. Epidemiology has demonstrated just how complex these interactions are. Thus, a cow that contracts an infection during the peripartum period runs a greater risk of contracting other diseases. Peripartum diseases are not isolated processes but rather a group of diseases that should be evaluated as a whole when deciding upon prevention and control strategies.

Throughout this book, we show, using descriptions of actual clinical cases, that peripartum diseases generally occur due to deviations from protocol, because the farmer does not follow the practical advice of the veterinary surgeon or is unfamiliar with the behavioural patterns of the cows. The cases described here will help the reader to appreciate that the causes underlying a complex cascade of peripartum disorders are often hard to find, but usually easy to treat.

As a clinician, the veterinary surgeon is responsible for the diagnosis and treatment of diseases, but must also be able to anticipate problems, and thus needs to be "proactive" rather than "reactive". The keys to achieving this goal are good management of data generated on the farm and proper interpretation of the clinical signs observed during inspection visits. During the peripartum period, the clinician cannot afford to wait for data to be generated in order to find solutions. Early diagnosis of herd diseases is the best approach to be able to implement the appropriate measures before problems arise.

This book describes the steps that must be taken between the time that a cow stops giving milk and peak lactation, using on-farm indicators that provide important information as to the welfare of the herd. This is a dynamic process involving the interaction of multiple factors. Our goal is to enable the reader to establish a decision tree with which to generate standard operating procedures.

2

Drying-off

Physiology

During the stage known as the dry period, the mammary gland first undergoes physiological atrophy, and then, in parallel with signs of approaching calving, undergoes hormone-mediated hypertrophy. In the case of an L1 (first lactation) cow experiencing its first dry period, mammogenesis will also occur. For practical purposes, dry periods should last for about 60 days to allow L1 cows to fully complete mammogenesis. As the calving date approaches, mammary hypertrophy becomes more evident and colostrum accumulates. The composition of colostrum differs significantly from that of the milk that is subsequently produced, containing twice as much calcium, 10 times more vitamin A, three times more vitamin D and 15 times more iron. Colostrum is in fact an immunoglobulin concentrate that immunises and protects calves. However, colostrum contains up to nine times the calcium concentration of circulating blood, and thus removes large amounts of calcium from the blood supply, resulting in significant bone loss by the female. During the dry period, the abdominal volume of the pregnant cow increases significantly; from the seventh month of pregnancy until calving, the foetus grows from 60 cm to 100 cm and its weight increases from approximately 15 kg to 35-40 kg (Table 1). By the end of the dry period, the ingestion capacity of the female is significantly limited, resulting in immunosuppression and increased susceptibility to changes. Appropriate handling is essential at this critical time (see Case 4, p. 114).

Table 1. Foetal development during the dry period.

	Months of gestation		
Foetal development during the dry period	7	8	9
Length	63 cm	80 cm	100 cm
Weight	15 kg	25 kg	40-50 kg

Drying-off: Why?

The start of the dry period corresponds to the end of one phase of lactation and preparatory stage of the subsequent phase. This constitutes an important rest period for the mammary gland. During the dry period, the udder undergoes involution and secretory cells are regenerated. The dry period can be viewed as a short-term investment: during this time it is important to carry out all planned or recommended management activities without delay.

Drying-off: When?

The duration of the dry period is determined relative to the calving interval, which should be evaluated in each case. Very long periods of lactation accompanied by prolonged dry periods often indicate reproductive failure, and are usually accompanied by postpartum conditions and an increase in body condition score. Table 2 shows the relative duration of the dry period with respect to the calving interval. While values can oscillate between 10 % and 18 %, the ideal range is between 12 % and 15 %.

As the dry period is a non-productive phase, it is desirable to minimise its duration.

The ideal duration is 45 to 65 days.

When deciding when to begin drying-off, it is important to consider the limiting factors that affect this process:

- **Stage of gestation and expected calving date:** these are factors that cannot be modified. The dry period should last a minimum of 45 days, or 60 days in the case of an L1 cow.
- **Production of milk before drying-off:** cows that show a sharp decline in milk production should be considered as candidates for drying-off, regardless of the stage of pregnancy. Ration cost and the body condition of the female should also be considered. Decreases in production are usually due to reproductive failure, which unnecessarily lengthens the lactation period, although other possible causes include mastitis, acute lameness, and a range of diverse diseases.
- **Body condition:** it is essential to evaluate this parameter. The ideal body condition score of a cow during the dry period is between 3 and 3.5. The female's body condition score should remain stable throughout the dry period. It is important to routinely monitor and comprehensively assess the body condition of cows on a farm, as this information will help determine the approach to be taken in cases where intervention is required. The milk conversion rate decreases at the end of the lactation period; if this change is accompanied by an increase in body condition score, the postpartum period will be negatively affected. Action is also required if a female shows signs of entering the dry period but produces more than the average yield of milk. We recommend drawing up a table, with the help of the farmer, and developing a routine of scoring the body condition and daily milk production of cows in the final stage of lactation.

Table 2. Relative duration of the dry period with respect to the calving interval.

Calving interval (days)	Dry period (days)		
	50	60	70
365	13.7 %	16.4 %	19.2 %
395	12.7 %	15.2 %	17.7 %
425	11.8 %	14.1 %	16.5 %
455	11.0 %	13.2 %	15.4 %

CONSIDERATIONS BEFORE DRYING-OFF

- What is the minimum physiologically appropriate dry period for the cow?
- Is it a first-lactation cow?
- What is the body condition score of the cow?
- Does the cow belong to a low-yield batch?
- Does the cow have a history of clinical or subclinical mastitis?
- What is the cow's somatic cell count?
- How many times did this cow have clinical mastitis during the last lactation?

By including additional data such as calving interval (days) and the duration (in days) of the dry period in this table, females can be effectively monitored and potential problems detected as soon as they arise. Adopting this routine in successive lactations provides a means of monitoring animals that are susceptible to disorders caused by poor body condition.

Drying-off: How?

Recommendations prior to the dry period:

- Always begin drying-off on the same day of the week.
- Modify the diet before drying-off to lower the energy content of the ration. This change is easily implemented when the concentrate is distributed automatically, but entails more difficult handling and increased stress to the animal in cases of manual distribution. Usually, alterations in the energy content of the ration are made when moving cows for drying-off from the lactation area.
- The change in diet should be implemented abruptly, but without altering milking. Before drying-off, the clinical history of each individual cow should be considered in consultation with a milk-quality vet, and treatment during the dry period should be protocolised as much as possible.
- **Healthy cows are treated with antibiotics upon drying-off** to prevent infection during the dry period and while calving.
- **Cows that are infected at the start of dry period** can be classified into three categories:
    - **Subclinical mastitis:** cows whose last individual somatic cell count was over

Dry cows should be housed in facilities that ensure a low-stress environment.

200,000 and in which the affected quarter has been identified in the CMT (California mastitis test). In these cases, samples should be taken for microbiological analyses, and treatment determined according to the pathogen isolated, as long as a selective antibiotic treatment is administered during the dry period.

- **Clinical mastitis:** this should be treated as described above for subclinical mastitis, although in this case a treatment is administered prior to the dry period antibiotic therapy.
- **Chronic mastitis:** these cows should receive specific treatment based on the results of the bacterial cultures during the last bouts of recurrent mastitis. This condition can be fully resolved by administering the appropriate treatment during the dry period.

Treatment failure during the dry period may result in:

- **Infected dry cows:** animals that are healthy before dry-off, but acquire mastitis during the dry period. Cows are at greatest risk of infection, mainly from gram-positive bacteria, 15 days before the atrophy of the mammary gland. There is an increased risk of gram-negative mastitis in the week before calving, which coincides with the hypertrophy of the mammary gland.
- **Cows infected after calving:** cows that are healthy during the dry period but present clinical or subclinical mastitis in early postpartum. These cows have individual somatic cell counts of over 200,000 in the first post-calving analysis. Although it is often assumed that many of these cows are infected during calving, they usually acquire infections during the dry period.

When a preventative antibiotic treatment is administered during the dry period, it should be done in conjunction with a cleaning and disinfection protocol, a proper use of medication, data traceability, and appropriate animal management.

Dry cow management

Drying-off entails a change to a different batch of cows (or two changes, if cows are fed a separate diet prior to drying-off) (Fig. 1). It is preferable that each of these adjustments is applied to more than one cow at a time, as this is less stressful for the animals concerned. The types of areas used for drying-off vary widely, and depend on several factors, such as the climate and the availability of space. For example, many farms on the Cantabrian coast, in the north of Spain, use old facilities that have been modified for this purpose (Fig. 2). Others fence off part of the milking area (usually without adequate aisles) for this purpose (Figs. 3 and 4), or use outdoor areas in all but the coldest winter months (Fig. 5). Animals that remain on pasture during the dry period should be checked daily for lameness and to monitor rumen content and udder condition. If animals are housed indoors, spacious, dry, well-ventilated facilities with a comfortable bed should be provided, and should be disinfected regularly. While the feeding area should be well illuminated, the remaining area need not be particularly bright, as darkness promotes the expression of prolactin receptors during the dry period (feedback effect). However, it is essential for milk production that the cow is housed in a well-lit area after calving (Fig. 6).

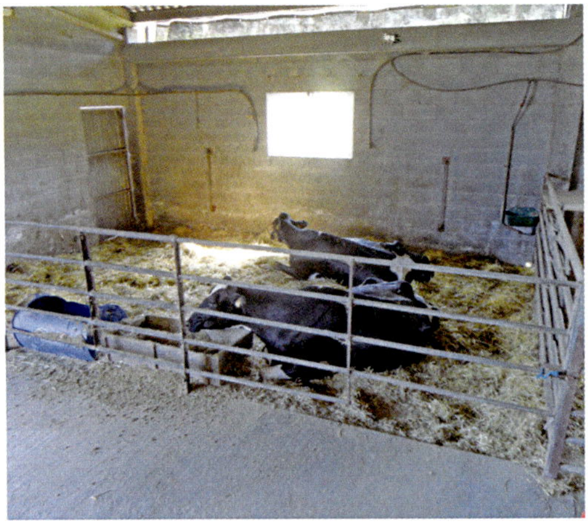

Figure 1. On some small farms, cows are separated from the main herd and fed a pre-drying-off diet before being moved to the dry cow batch.

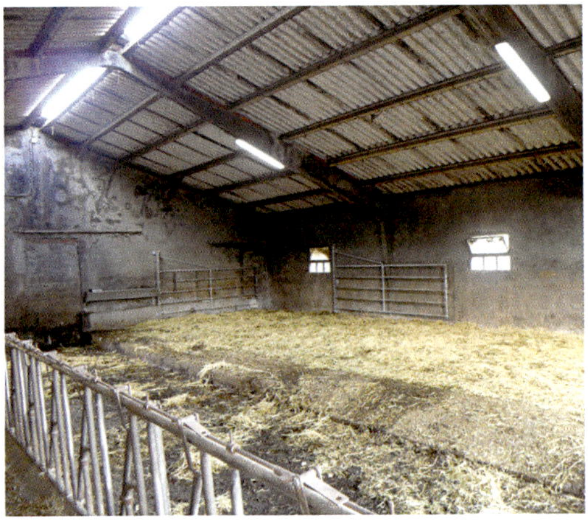

Figure 2. Old farmhouse adapted for drying-off. Note how one of the corridors has been filled in with concrete to eliminate the step and provide a space to lay the bedding. In the background is a simple gating system used to fence off the calving area.

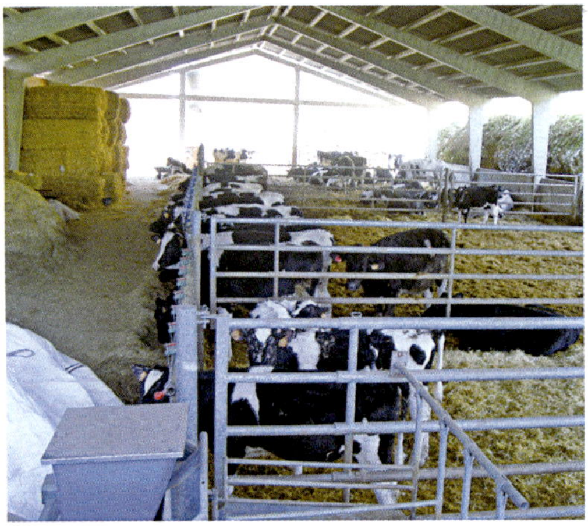

Figure 3. Intensive farm with separate pens for rearing and for dry cows (background).

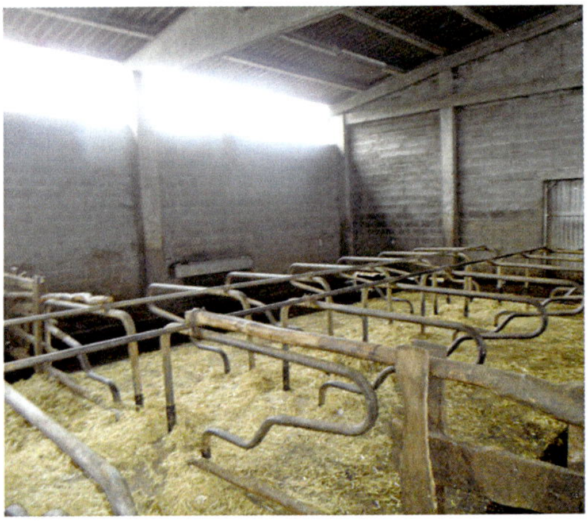

Figure 4. Area within the milking facility used to house dry cows. Despite the blind corridor, the space is adequate (with the necessary beds, water troughs, etc.).

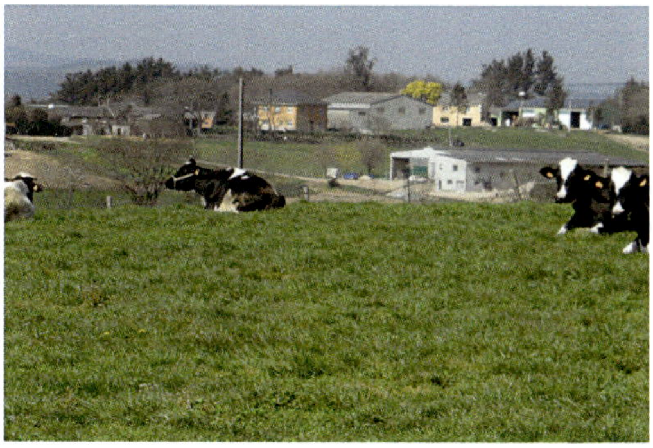

Figure 5. On the oceanic climatic areas, dry cows usually remain in the fields in good weather. This may be most of the year, except for the harshest winter months.

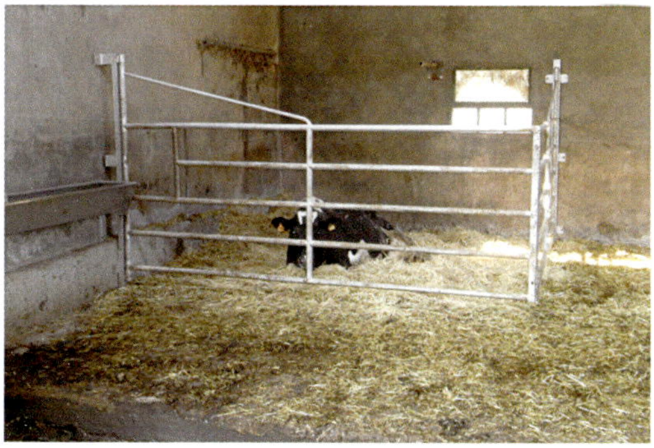

Figure 6. Area used as a calving pen. Note the bed and water trough.

Treatments that can be applied during the dry period

Podiatric treatments

Any injury to the legs of a dry cow, whether mechanical or infectious, should be tended to immediately. Cattle crushes have been continually modernised and improved, decreasing the risk to cows of abdominal compression. Moreover, the degree of stress induced by occasional handling will be always less than that caused by a limp that becomes permanent or recurrent due to a failure to treat on time. Lame cows suffer pain and immobility, and are thus less well prepared to face the challenges of calving and lactation (see Cases 1 and 2, p. 106 and 108).

Vaccinations

Vaccination protocols established by farming associations can be applied during the dry period, and vaccinations against mastitis in the dam and viral diarrhoea in the future offspring can be administered. It may also be of interest to vaccinate against certain respiratory processes, such as bovine respiratory syncitial virus (BRSV), *Parainfluenza* 3 (PI3), and *Pasteurella*, to revaccinate against enterotoxaemias, ringworm or leptospirosis, among other diseases, and to administer other injectable treatments during the dry period. The aim of these treatments is to immunise the offspring and to protect the mother against any processes that may jeopardise her health during the critical postpartum period.

Antiparasitic treatments

There are as many antiparasitic protocols as there are indications for their use. If cows are kept outside during the dry period, they run an increased risk of parasitisation, especially if the dry period coincides with spring and summer. In any grazing area, the amount and variety of endoparasites should be controlled to some degree. Wet areas represent a particular threat, and a previously established prevention protocol should be applied to cows grazing in this type of area, independent of the results of periodic stool analysis (Figs. 7 and 8).

Some ectoparasites such as ticks can transmit serious and fatal diseases such as piroplasmosis (babesiosis and theileriosis) and anaplasmosis. These diseases can manifest as acute outbreaks, usually in cows that are dried off outdoors in spring time (see Case 6, p. 126). Cows should also be checked for scabies mites and lice so that they can be treated as soon as they appear, and should be monitored for filariasis, which often causes ulcer-like lesions around the udder, and can be complicated by fungal processes (Fig. 9). In any event, the dry period is a good time to attempt to cure an infected animal, as milk production will not be interrupted by the treatment.

Other preventative treatments

The prevention protocols of each farm vary depending on the types of diseases most commonly encountered. Preventative treatments include vitamin supplements (A, D3, E), selenium, propylene glycol (around the time of calving), lipotropic substances (for cows with high body condition scores), and amino acids.

BODY CONDITION ASSESSMENT

The body condition of cows should be routinely assessed and those with increased risk of variation should be monitored closely. Ideally, cows should be grouped according to body condition during the dry period.

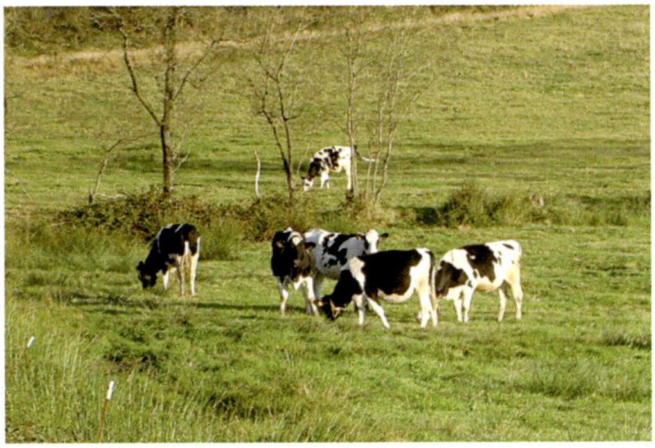

Figure 7. On many farms, calves and dry cows share areas with high parasite loads. The presence of reeds in this case indicates that the animals are grazing in a very wet area.

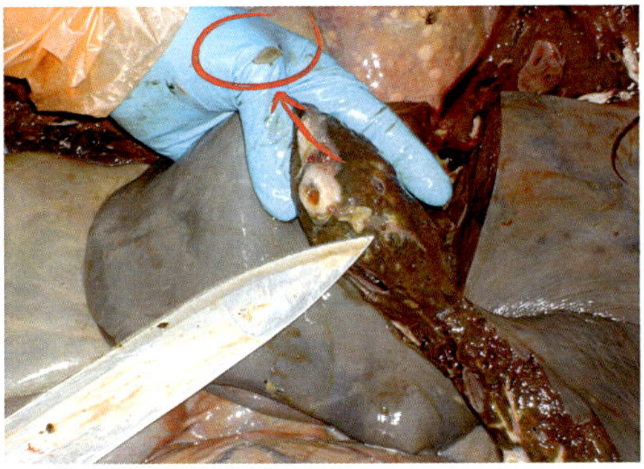

Figure 8. Fasciolosis. Animals kept in wet meadows are parasitised at a higher rate.

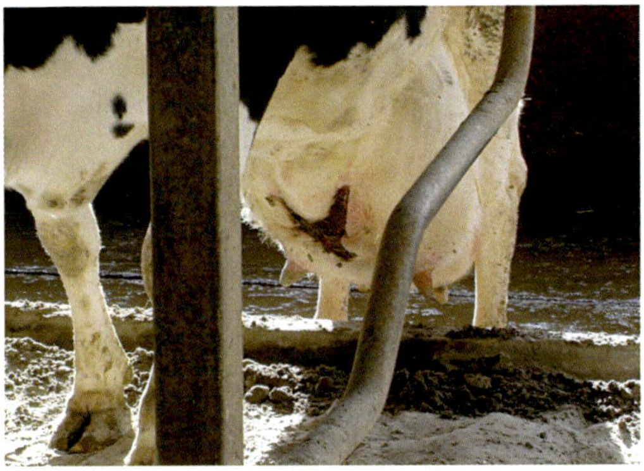

Figure 9. Typical lesion caused by filarial parasites; usually these injuries are complicated by the appearance of fungi. During the dry period, topical and antiparasitic treatments can be applied.

3

Late pregnancy and calving

During pregnancy, foetal development can be altered by diseases of the mother, including conditions that cause miscarriage or mummification, accidents, or particularly stressful circumstances (e.g. construction on the farm, noise, storms, sanitation operations, or mass vaccinations, such as the first vaccination against bluetongue).

Table 1 in Chapter 2 (see p. 6) shows the increase in the size and weight of the foetus from seven months of gestation until calving.

Increasingly, veterinary surgeons are required to confirm pregnancy by rectal examination before drying-off. In other cases, vets are required to evaluate pregnancy-related diseases, regardless of the stage of gestation.

Pregnancy monitoring before drying-off

During routine check-ups, the veterinary surgeon should first verify the available data for each pregnant cow and establish a work plan based on the scheduled dates of subsequent examinations. The quality of the available data should be assessed as some information may be missing or incorrect.

Late pregnancy examination

When rectally examining a cow between months five and seven of gestation, the following signs should be evaluated:

1. The first anatomical point of reference is the **cervix**. The pregnant uterus offers inherent resistance when gently pulled towards a caudal position, allowing the veterinary surgeon to assess its contents. The uterus descends towards the abdominal cavity, where it can be examined by the vet. The relative relaxation of the uterine wall can be assessed, and the cotyledons palpated with the fingertips to determine their size and diameter.

   In some cases, foetal vitality can be assessed by direct palpation, regardless of the stage of gestation. However, even in late gestation (5-7 months) **it may be impossible to palpate the foetus**, which may be located deep in the abdominal cavity, at least at the moment of examination. This can be surprising to the farmer and frustrating for the vet.
2. **The ovaries maintain their anatomical position throughout gestation, and are thus accessible** at all times. The ovary of the gravid horn can be distinguished from the contralateral ovary by the presence of the corpus luteum. While the difference between the two ovaries can be easily appreciated by ultrasound, some practice is required to distinguish one from the other by palpation.
3. Finally, the vet should examine **the uterine arteries**, which can be easily located between 3.5 and 4 months of gestation. The uterine artery that supplies the gravid uterine horn can be felt in the broad ligament, through which it runs. It is important to palpate these structures gently, as they may go unnoticed if excessive pressure is applied (Fig. 1). The veterinary surgeon will note the pulse of the arteries.

The number of indicators and parameters to be assessed and analysed increases as pregnancy progresses.

The artery supplying the non-gravid uterine horn also increases in diameter and can be palpated between 5.5 and 6 months of gestation, although this artery will always be smaller than that corresponding to the gravid horn. Both uterine arteries should be examined.

We recommend beginning the pregnancy examination by palpating the ovaries to first identify that which corresponds to the gravid uterine horn, and then palpating the artery that supplies this horn. Care should be taken to avoid any errors during the examination, as these can result in miscalculation of the dry-off date.

Remember, if only the uterine artery corresponding to the non-gravid horn is palpated, the

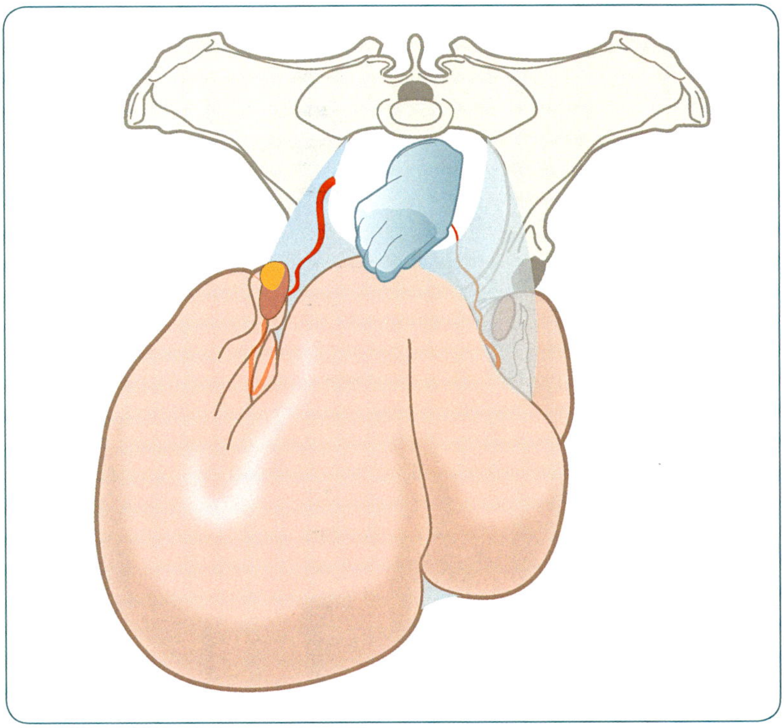

Figure 1. Seven months of gestation. The uterine arteries that run through the broad ligaments of the uterus can be palpated during the rectal examination.

> As a rule of thumb, the gravid and non-gravid uterine arteries can be differentiated by palpation after six months of gestation.

stage of gestation can be underestimated by two months. If it is possible to palpate both arteries, it should be borne in mind that the relationship between the arteries of the pregnant and non-gravid uterine horns is as follows:

Artery supplying gravid uterine horn	Artery supplying non-gravid uterine horn
6 months	4 months
7 months	5 months
8 months	6 months
9 months	7 months

For this reason, caution is advised when diagnosing pregnancy in cases in which both uterine arteries cannot be adequately palpated, or when the available data are insufficient to confirm the status or stage of gestation. The initial diagnosis can always be revised at a later date.

For example, if correct data are not available or if the examination is not correctly performed, a cow that is 7.5 months pregnant may appear to be just over 5 months pregnant. This can result in the cow not being dried off at the right time, or erroneously suggest a problem with the pregnancy, thus leading to incorrect decisions.

In some cases, twin pregnancies can also give rise to confusion, especially if not detected when the pregnancy is first diagnosed. In these cases, two corpora lutea develop in the same or in different ovaries. When the two foetuses are contained within one uterine horn, the artery supplying the gravid horn may have a larger than normal diameter. By contrast, both horns are usually of a similar diameter when each contains one foetus. These features can lead to confusion when evaluating the stage of gestation. Measurement of artery diameter is highly subjective, and this value is thus not worth quantifying. Moreover, the ease with which the arteries can be palpated will depend on the body condition and fatness of the cow. When it comes to performing the pregnancy examination, exceptions and difficulties can always arise, such as uterine adhesions from previous caesareans, abscesses and fibroids. If a proper record-keeping protocol is followed, these abnormalities should already be recorded in the reproductive record of the animal. The vet should always perform pregnancy diagnoses while referring to the reproductive and medical history of the animal concerned.

Pregnancy-related disorders

The vet may also be required to attend to sick pregnant cows. Pregnancy-related conditions include foetal mummification, imminent miscarriage and prepartum uterine torsion.

Foetal mummification

The vet may encounter this type of condition upon performing a specific reproductive examination of a cow, or by chance during a routine visit to a farm.

Diagnosis

Depending on the stage of the mummification process, the first observation during rectal palpation is the relative ease with which the uterus can be lifted by gently retracting the cervix. In cases of foetal mummification, the uterus weighs less than normal due to fluid loss, the uterine wall is smoother and the cotyledons typical of a normal pregnancy cannot be felt. Often, the veterinary surgeon can directly touch the foetus (due to the absence of surrounding fluid), which lacks vital signs. Usually, the uterine artery supplying the gravid uterine horn is of a smaller diameter than expected, although some residual pulse may be detected.

Treatment

The situation should be assessed from an economic point of view, taking into account the days in milk, calving number, and genetic value, as well as potential infectious processes that may have caused the mummification.

When diagnosing pregnancy in a cow that has already reached mid-gestation, the information obtained by palpation of the foetus, ovaries and uterine arteries should be evaluated. This information is more reliable when supported by clinical history data and other available records.

If it is decided to slaughter the cow, the meat obtained can in principle be used for human consumption.

If it is decided to treat the cow and attempt to impregnate her once again, prostaglandins should be administered and the effects monitored. In some cases, the mummified foetus is small enough to become trapped in the vagina. Accordingly, the animal should be examined between two and five days after prostaglandin treatment. It may be necessary to repeat the treatment again after 10-15 days. Once treated, the cow should be impregnated again as soon as possible.

Imminent miscarriage

Usually, a farmer will contact a vet when a pregnant cow is behaving unusually, straining, or expelling fluid from the vagina, or when the foetus becomes visible.

Diagnosis

The possible causes of miscarriage are very diverse. Miscarriage may also be a sign of disease.

First, the veterinary surgeon should evaluate the general health of the animal. It is advisable to then perform a vaginal examination to determine the degree of dilation of the cervix and whether the foetus is in a dystocic position, in which case it should be repositioned. In the early stages of miscarriage, the cervix is usually closed. In these cases, rectal examination reveals an increased uterine tone and a tighter than normal uterine wall due to the increased release of prostaglandins associated with miscarriage. Foetal or uterine emphysema should also be evaluated; confirmation of either of these processes indicates an extreme case and a low likelihood of saving the life of the cow.

Treatment

Normally, cow meat obtained immediately after a miscarriage cannot be used for human consumption. Accordingly, the protocol followed in cases of miscarriage favours expulsion of the foetus, isolation and treatment of the cow and subsequent evaluation of the possibility of impregnating the cow once again. Additional factors that should be considered include the days in milk, calving number, and genetic value. A study of the possible causes of the miscarriage should also be conducted.

The generic treatment involves:

- Treatment with antibiotics and prostaglandins.
- Monitoring and examination of the cow every 6-8 hours, and extraction of the foetus if necessary.

In the event of foetal emphysema, the chances of treatment success are lower, and the vet often has to resort to foetal extraction, which is usually very laborious. In these cases, it is highly unlikely that the cow can become pregnant again and it may have to be sent to slaughter. A caesarean should only be performed if the uterine wall shows no signs of emphysema, as this entails a high risk of peritoneal contamination by both the foetus and contaminated fluids.

In short, the best approach is that which prioritises the survival of the mother, who can subsequently be sold and whose meat can be used after completion of the drug withdrawal period.

Prepartum uterine torsion

This type of condition can appear after 7 months of gestation, even though the cow may not yet be ready to calve.

Diagnosis

Uterine torsion is diagnosed by examination after evaluating the symptoms and medical history of the cow. Examination the cow usually reveals restlessness, loss of appetite, tachycardia, signs of pain, straining, signs of colic, and a sudden drop in production if the cow is still lactating.

After vaginal and rectal examination of the cow, the vet should be able to locate the site of the torsion:

- **Precervical torsion:** the torsion occurs between the contents of the uterus and the cervix. This situation causes foetal distress. The vagina and cervix can be relatively relaxed and in some cases diagnosis can be very difficult.
- **Postcervical torsion:** the torsion occurs after the cervix and clearly affects the vagina. The cervical entrance deviates towards the side of the torsion and the tension causes the formation of vaginal folds.

> The extent to which blood flow is impaired and the clinical signs depend on the degree of uterine torsion.

For the same degree of uterine torsion, the viability of both the mother and foetus is greater in cases of postcervical versus precervical torsion.

While postcervical torsion can be diagnosed by **vaginal examination**, precervical torsion may go unnoticed.

Both precervical and postcervical torsion can be diagnosed by **rectal examination**. This is the most reliable method for detecting precervical torsion, as the tension of the uterine ligaments (broad ligaments) can be properly appreciated. Moreover, rectal examination provides an indication of the degree of torsion, and of possible emphysema of the foetus or the uterine wall.

Treatment

This section discusses some possible solutions to uterine torsion, but does not describe a treatment per se for this particular condition. The likelihood of successfully treating uterine torsion in a cow that is not calving is always low (poor prognosis). It is important to first inform the farmer and the personnel involved of the situation.

- The cow should not be rolled if it is not yet calving, as the foetus cannot be adequately grabbed or pulled.
- Restorative laparotomy is the only solution. However, this approach should only be employed when the torsion is diagnosed at an early stage and no visible alterations to the uterus are observed. Definitive resolution of the problem is not possible, and thus the best possible outcome is correction of the torsion (Fig. 2). This surgery is not without complications due to the risks associated with uterine and foetal manipulation. During the surgical procedure, foetal vitality should be assessed; this allows the vet to decide whether to extract the foetus by caesarean section (if dead) (Fig. 3). The farmer should always be advised in advance of the possible risks of surgery.
- If the vet identifies factors that have clearly caused the torsion (e.g. lameness, confined enclosures that prevent the animal from comfortably raising itself from the ground), the best option is to use the cow for its meat (relevant legislation permitting).
- The veterinary surgeon should try to correct the uterine torsion by laparotomy until total relaxation of the ligaments and vessels is observed. Finally, antibiotics should be administered, shock should be prevented, and the animal should be allowed time to rest and recover.

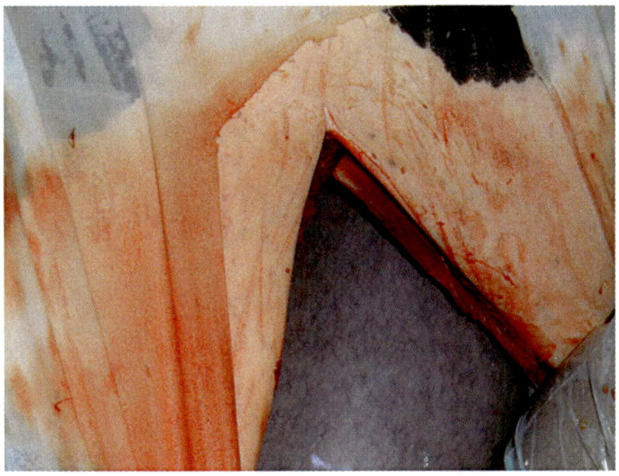

Figure 2. Cow with precervical uterine torsion before calving (eight months of gestation). Cyanosis of the uterus (gravid horn) due to impaired arterial and venous circulation can be observed. In this case, the vet decided to perform a caesarean section in order to save the cow.

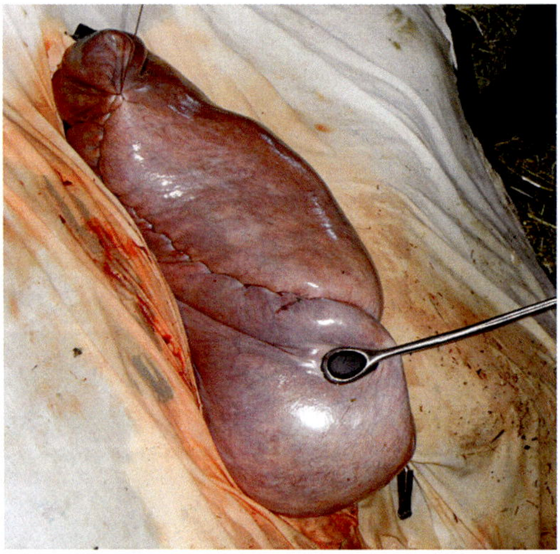

Figure 3. Caesarean section after resolution of uterine torsion. Note the return of blood flow to the uterine wall (see Fig. 2), although the serosa has not yet regained its normal appearance.

Calving

Milk production begins after calving. This is a tense time for both farmers and vets, as it marks the end of one phase and the beginning of another, and the outcome determines the success of the entire productive phase of the cow in both heifers and multiparous females. It takes a lot of work to bring a cow to calving in good health and the management of this crucial period significantly influences the lactation curve of the cow (Fig. 4). The highest percentage of diseases occurs during the peripartum period.

Physiological calving

Hormonal changes

Levels of **progesterone**, which are maintained during pregnancy by secretions from the placenta and ovaries, drop sharply a few hours before calving.

Oestrogen levels increase gradually throughout gestation, but a more pronounced rise occurs in the last week of gestation, with levels peaking two days before delivery. Oestrogen promotes the development of the myometrium and the synthesis of actomyosin, which facilitates uterine contractions during calving. These hormones are also involved in the relaxation of the bony joints of the birth canal of the cow, promoting elasticity and preparing the pelvis for calving.

Approximately 24 hours before calving, interactions between the foetus and placenta, changes in the myometrium and the progressive increase in oestrogen levels trigger a cascade of hormonal events that increase the concentrations of **corticosteroids** and **prolactin** (Fig. 5). In turn, these two hormones stimulate increased production of the **natural prostaglandins relaxin** and **oxytocin**, which facilitate calving.

Stages of calving

Preparation (duration: 2-8 hours)

The preparation phase involves the final hormonal changes, which occur in the last 24 hours before expulsion of the foetus. The cow may appear restless, especially if it is not in its usual surroundings. Pregnant animals are highly sensitive to changes in surroundings, companions, and personnel.

Dilation (duration: 2-6 hours)

During this phase, uterine contractions begin and the foetus turns or alters its position in order to advance through the birth canal; the foetus is usually already inclined within the uterus before dilation begins. The foetus rotates and stretches its head and limbs within the amniotic and allantoic sacs, orientating itself towards the birth

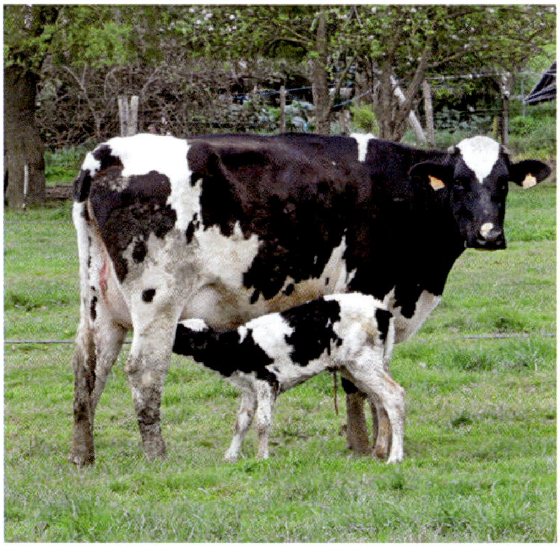

Figure 4. Fresh cow with her calf suckling colostrum, both in good health.

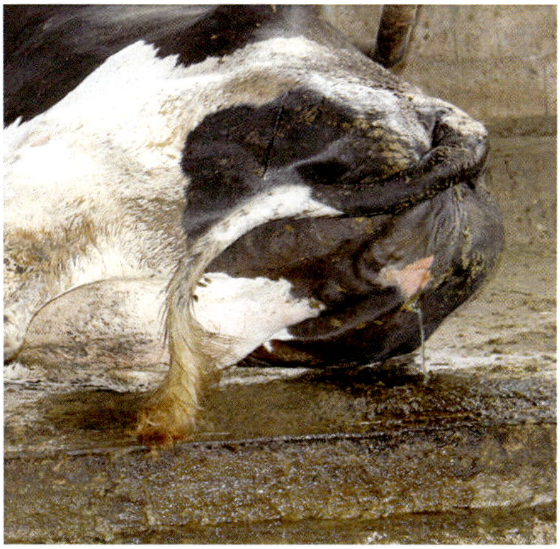

Figure 5. Cow in the prepartum period. Calving will take place within 36 hours.

canal. The cervix adopts a wedge-like shape that accommodates the head, the hooves of the forelimbs and other adjacent structures of the calf, and progressively dilates and opens from the uterus towards the vagina, ultimately forming a single channel linking the uterus, cervix and vagina.

In primiparous cows, even in cases of a vaginal delivery, the final portion of this channel slightly impedes the exit of the foetus, as the vaginal vestibule is usually less elastic than in multiparous females.

Note that posterior presentation of the foetus diminishes the "wedge effect" of the calf's head against the cervix. In practice, posterior presentation is often interpreted as a dystocia. Foetal vitality is reduced in these cases; the umbilical cord usually ruptures in an abnormal manner, and vaginal peritoneum is scarce. In these cases, there is an increased risk of patent urachus, which results in damaged blood vessels and can give rise to infection. Veterinary assistance with calving is more often required in cases of posterior versus anterior presentation, and the extraction technique is more complicated.

Foetal expulsion (duration: 0.5-2 hours)

During this stage, the foetus completes its rotation in the uterus and moves towards the cervix. The presence of the calf in the birth canal has a stimulatory effect on the intensity and frequency of the cow's contractions. The stretching movements of the foetus, which begin during dilation, now involve the hindlimbs (anterior presentation). These movements of the hindlimbs are probably responsible for the appearance of abscesses, adhesions and parametritis, which are sometimes detected in the postpartum examination, even in healthy cows that required no assistance during calving and did not experience placental retention or metritis.

SIGNS OF LABOUR

Hormonal changes cause certain physical alterations that appear during a normal delivery:

- Vulvar, perineal or mammary oedema (Fig. 6).
- Relaxation of the pelvic muscles and the pubic symphysis, which softens the birth canal and eases the passage of the foetus.
- This change, together with the descent of the foetus, gives the abdomen a pear-like shape and results in the relaxation of the hip muscles.
- Dilation of the teat cistern. This change is often easiest appreciated in multiparous females, as in primiparous cows it may be obscured due to oedema. This clinical sign indicates that the cow will calve in less than 12 hours.

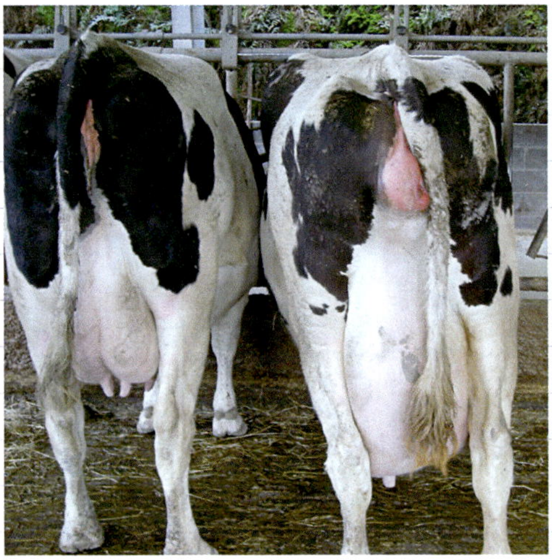

Figure 6. Prepartum oedema of the vulva and udder. This cow has been lying on its right side, and thus the oedema is more evident on the left side.

In any case, all the typical clinical signs of calving should be assessed as a whole.

Normally, the allantoic and amniotic sacs protrude before the foetus. These sacs are ruptured by vulvar pressure and by the contractions of the cow, although in some cases they must be manually ruptured, particularly the amniotic sac. In other cases, these sacs can rupture within the uterus; this phenomenon is almost always associated with dystocia.

Except in cases of dystocia, free-standing cows always lie down prior to expulsion of the foetus. In this position, the abdominal muscles work effectively and the hip is firmly supported by the ground. The pubic symphysis of the cow is separated by the action of hormones at the time of calving, decreasing the stability of the hip.

The side on which lies the cow is important for successful calving. Before the cow begins calving (physiological, anterior presentation), the foetus will be slightly inclined within the uterus to either the right or left; the cow will lie down on the side towards which the foetus is inclined, such that the spinal columns of dam and calf are parallel. This position favours the lateral advancement of the head of the foetus towards the sacrum, avoiding the sacral ridge, and allows maximum use of the full width of the birth canal. The same occurs in cases of posterior presentation: the buttocks of the calf enter the birth canal obliquely. When assisting this type of delivery, traction should be alternately applied to each of the hind limbs, moving one buttock forward and then the other. It is important that the female is lying down when performing this kind of manipulation, as this decreases the risk of dislocating the hip.

Expulsion of the foetus takes longer in primiparous cows, due to the narrowness of the vaginal opening.

Expulsion of the placenta (duration: 2-12 hours)

Calving does not end until the placenta is delivered. Until this happens, personnel assisting the cow should remain vigilant, keep the surroundings clean and handle the cow with care (Fig. 7).

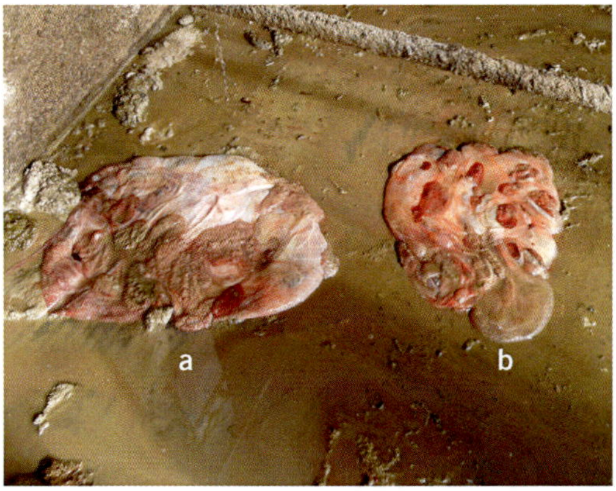

Figure 7. Unusual case of placental expulsion. The placenta of the gravid uterine horn (a) can be distinguished from that of the non-gravid horn (b). Note the differences in the size and diameter of the cotyledons of the two uterine horns.

The length of this phase can vary greatly, as evidenced by the highly variable data presented in the bibliography; any dystocia or concurrent disease can influence the delivery of the placenta. This phase begins hours before the expulsion of the foetus, with the hormonal changes of the preparatory phase, which induces physiological ischaemia of the attachments between the cotyledons and caruncles.

Puerperium (early postpartum)

Uterine involution begins once the foetal membranes have been expelled; within 24 hours the cervix is almost closed and within 4-6 days uterine size is reduced by half. A few hours after calving, the cow expels the remaining fluids (lochia) from the amniotic and allantoic sacs. From this point on, these emissions become less frequent. Lochia consist of exudates and the remnants of cotyledons, and are mainly expelled between postpartum days 10 and 12. These excretions are turbid and may vary in colour (depending on the presence or absence of metritis). The colour and texture of the lochia can vary considerably if the cow has a concurrent infection. When postpartum cows are in good health, the uterus should exhibit good muscle tone.

This period is very important; many studies have proposed a relationship between the progression of milk production in the first days after calving and future productive and reproductive rates of the cow.

Indications for calving

- **Avoid changes in handling when calving is imminent.** Any change in the handling of the cow can be stressful, and more so if it occurs close to the time of calving. For this reason,

TYPES OF LOCHIA

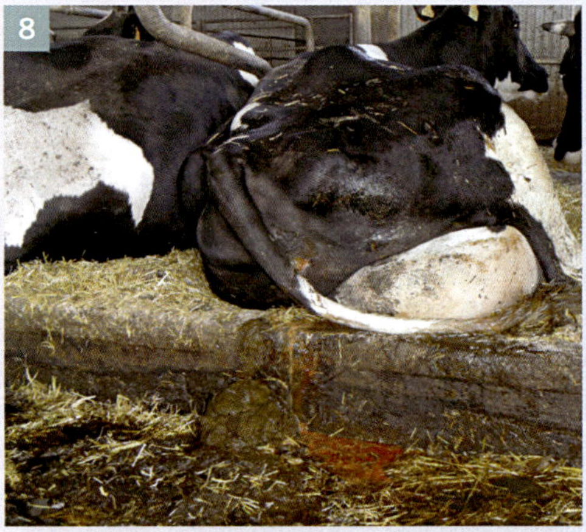

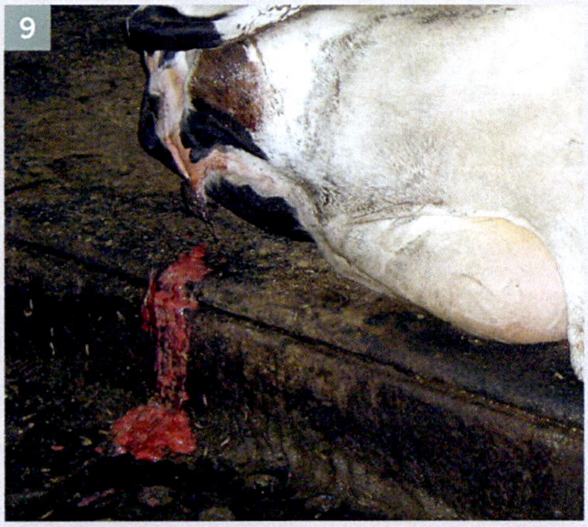

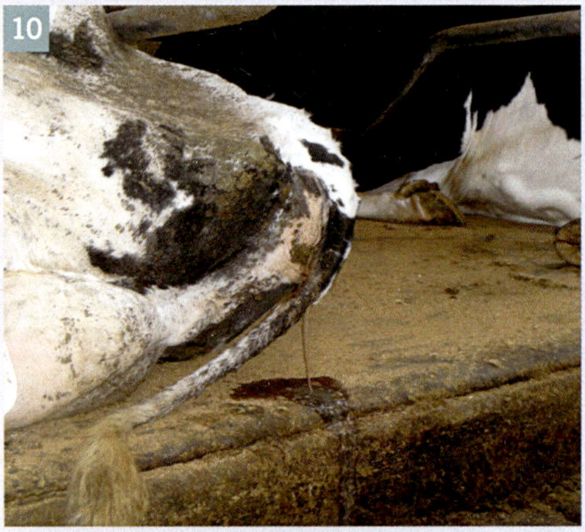

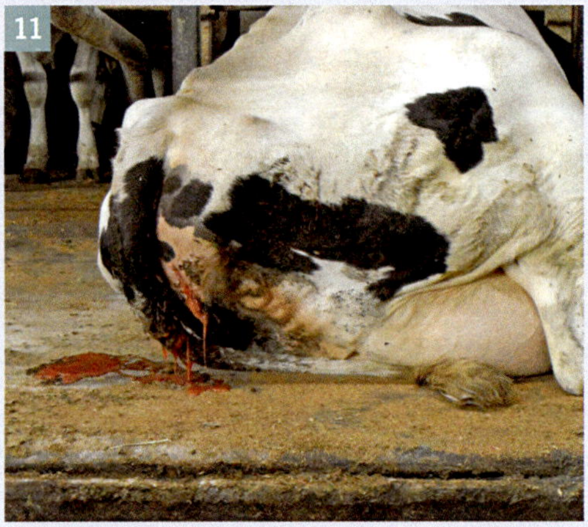

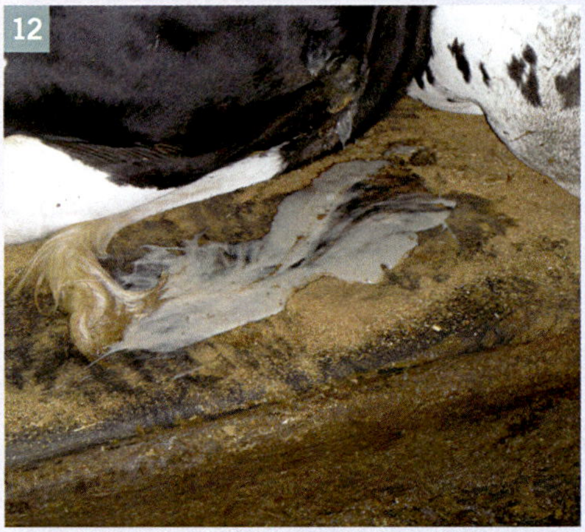

Figure 8. Cow expelling lochia three days after calving.

Figure 9. Cow three days after calving, expelling dense lochia containing traces of blood.

Figure 10. Cow nine days after calving, expelling healthy looking, relatively thin and clean lochia.

Figure 11. Cow 10 days after calving, expelling dense lochia containing traces of blood.

Figure 12. Cow 11 days after calving, expelling whitish lochia (metritis).

REMEMBER

It is important to carefully monitor the cow during the early postpartum period. This is a critical and delicate time from both the physiological and financial point of view in terms of future productivity. Better management of the postpartum cow allows the establishment of more effective preventative or remedial measures, ultimately increasing the animal's profitability.

batches should be established according to certain criteria to avoid the need for major physical or social disruption during this period. These measures ensure that the cow can calve in familiar surroundings. Nearby facilities can be used for the moment of calving, but social disruption should be avoided. Remember that calving does not end until the cow expels the placenta.

- **It is important to monitor the cow and assist during calving if necessary.** Calving should take place somewhere that allows easy monitoring by personnel, without unnecessary disturbance of the cow. Hasty or excessive manipulations should be avoided.
- **The calving area must be clean.** The area in which the cow calves should be clean, spacious, comfortable and safe (non-slip floor), and should be appropriately prepared to see to the needs of the neonatal calf. If the cow requires assistance while calving, suitable, clean materials (e.g. calving ropes, lubricants) should always be used, and clean water should be available. The use of household oils or detergents is not recommended.

Dystocia

Any factor that alters the normal physiology of calving can trigger a dystocia.

Problems of the mother or foetus as causes of dystocia

Disproportionate foetus

In the case of an obvious disparity in the size of the foetus, the veterinary surgeon should evaluate the situation and decide whether to perform a forced extraction or a caesarean. When a disproportionate foetus has difficulties entering the birth canal, a caesarean section is always the best option. If the calf is subjected to strong thoracic pressure during the passage through the maternal pelvis, it may experience significant foetal distress, resulting in very low viability. We recommend performing a higher percentage of caesarean sections than strictly necessary to avoid this potential outcome. Regardless of the value of the calf, poor decisions taken by the vet can also endanger the milk production of the cow.

Primiparous cows

It is not recommended to rush into manipulations of the foetus, even if the calf's hooves and snout

All stages of labour usually last longer in heifers than in multiparous cows.

are showing. However, it is important that the vet is vigilant. Sometimes, the foetus may need assistance in passing through the ring formed by the vestibule and the vulva. Usually, gentle traction using suitable materials is sufficient to extract the foetus. However, an episiotomy is recommended if there is a danger of perineal tearing. In many cases, sudden manipulations can result in functional alterations in the cow (e.g. loss of rigidity in the roof of the vaginal vestibule). This in turn can trigger perineal tears or conditions such as pneumovagina (see Cases 5.1 and 5.2, p. 117 and 121), which affect the recovery of the postpartum cow and even subsequent lactation. Moreover, problems that arise due to poor handling of calving heifers can result in infertility just when these animals should be beginning their productive phase, and before they have generated any economic return.

Posterior presentation

Calving can be considered dystocic when the foetus presents in the posterior position. The best possible outcome in these cases is that the birth canal receives the foetus in breech position. As compared with the anterior position, the pressure exerted by a foetus in posterior presentation upon the uterus is reduced.

Once the presentation of the foetus and the relationship between the longitudinal axes of the spinal columns of the mother and calf have been verified, it is recommended to cast the cow on the appropriate side and proceed with the extraction of the foetus. Ropes are often used to facilitate calving. A rope is tied to each limb and traction is alternately applied to advance the hips of the calf.

Foetal viability is lower in cases of posterior presentation as compared with anterior presentation. After calving, the calf should be placed in an upright position to facilitate clearing of the airways by gravity, independent of pharmacological support using cardiorespiratory analeptics.

Malpresentations

An entire book could be written on this topic alone. We recommend the "Pathological Calving" chapter in Franz Benesch's *Veterinary Obstetrics*.

The diagnosis of malpresentations and their treatment using pharmacological and surgical methods has improved greatly over the years. By contrast, the field of obstetrics continues to rely on principles that were described quite some time ago (Fig. 13).

Calving with uterine torsion

This type of dystocia is relatively common. The female is ready to calve, but dilation fails to

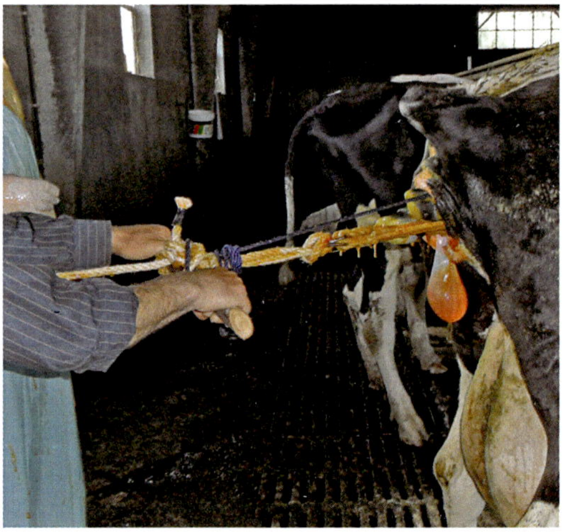

Figure 13. Dystocia due to malpresentation (flexion of the foetal head). This dystocia is corrected by securing the jaw of the calf with a rope with which the foetus is subsequently extracted.

progress and the foetus is not expelled. In some cases, torsion is diagnosed only hours before calving, and thus the cow cannot dilate or expel the foetus as it is not hormonally prepared at the time of calving.

Aetiology

The causes of uterine torsion vary widely:

- Confinement or inadequately-sized cubicles. Cows have less space in which to stand up, which sometimes requires multiple attempts.
- Different types of lameness, especially forelimb injuries. This type of lameness causes the cow to support itself on its knees and to rock from side to side in this position for some time before standing up (Fig. 14).
- Transport of cows close to the date of calving.
- Sudden movements of the foetus during calving.
- Presence of bulls in batches of dry cows. The males can stress newly arrived females, who may feel threatened.

Symptoms

Cows with a uterine torsion may present different clinical manifestations, e.g. milk ejection, filled teat cistern, and signs of discomfort (frequently rising and lying back down) (Figs. 15 and 16). The cow may also strain and elevate the base of its tail and is often colicky (striking itself on the abdomen with its head or one of its legs).

Diagnosis

To diagnose uterine torsion, it is essential to know:

- **If the cow is calving**

  Data on artificial insemination or natural mating should be obtained in advance, and signs of calving should be assessed.

  On performing a vaginal examination, the veterinary surgeon will be able to determine the extent to which access to the uterus is impaired, which in turn indicates the degree of torsion. Hormonal activity at the time of calving

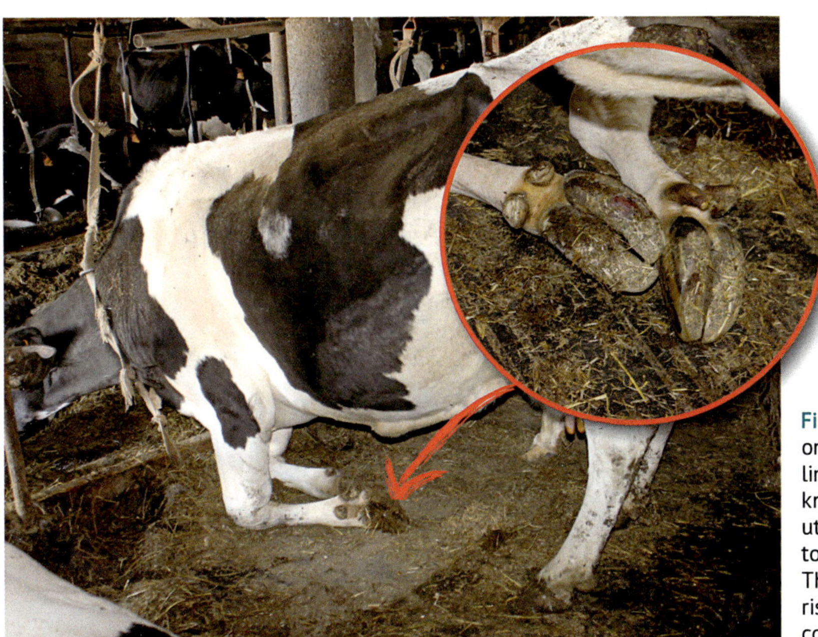

Figure 14. Cow with ulcers on the hooves of the forelimbs. The animal remains kneeling for several minutes and rocks from side to side before getting up. This situation increases the risk of torsion in pregnant cows.

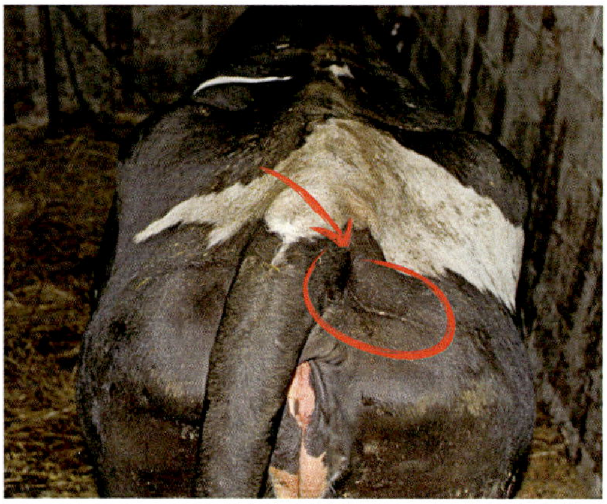

Figure 15. Calving cow with dystocia due to anti-clock-wise uterine torsion (viewed from the rear). Note the depression on the right side of the cow due to increased tension of the ligaments and muscles of the uterus caused by the rotation.

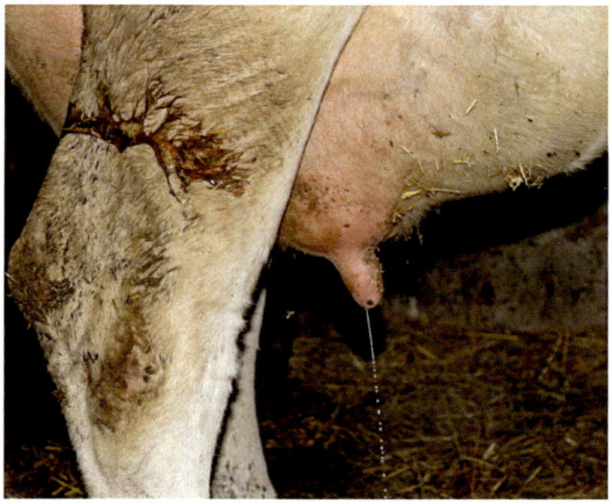

Figure 16. Expulsion of milk. This may occur in dystocias that prolong calving.

softens the tissue and facilitates the vet's access to the uterus, even in cases of uterine torsion, provided that they pass the vaginal folds and rotate the hand accordingly.

- **Extent and direction of torsion**
  - **Precervical torsion:** this torsion occurs at the highest part of the uterus, before the cervix. This type of torsion poses the greatest risk to the lives of the mother and calf, because it reduces the space available to the foetus in utero. Compared with other types of torsion, the same degree of precervical torsion has a more detrimental effect on blood circulation. Precervical torsion is also more difficult to diagnose; if no major displacement of the cervix occurs it may go unnoticed in a vaginal examination, and thus it is essential to check for torsion rectally. It is important to determine the direction of the torsion (clockwise or anticlockwise, as viewed from behind) for proper resolution, regardless of the method used.
  - **Postcervical torsion:** this type of torsion occurs posterior to the cervix and also affects the vagina, and thus is more easily diagnosed by vaginal examination. To reach the uterus during a vaginal examination the vet must rotate his/her hand (like a corkscrew) and follow the direction of the rotation. The vaginal arteries are located on the floor of the vagina. Postcervical torsion can result in the displacement of these arteries; in cases of torsion to the left, the right vaginal right artery will be elevated due to the rotation of the uterus (and vice versa in the case of torsion to the right). Depending on the degree of rotation, access to the uterus can be impaired, and thus a rectal examination is advised.
- **The degree of torsion**

  Uterine torsion can involve varying degrees of rotation (90°, 180° and 270°), which can block vaginal access to the uterus and impede resolution. In cases of 90° rotations, the uterus can usually be easily accessed via the cervix, and this type of torsion, even when diagnosed only hours before delivery, can self-resolve due to the movements of the mother and foetus during the preparatory phase. In any case, the greater the degree of rotation, the greater the impairment of circulation of both the mother and foetus and the more difficult it is to resolve. Vaginal and rectal examinations can indicate the level of tension in ligaments (Fig. 17) and allow the vet to determine the degree of torsion, although such interpretations are always subjective.

Treatment

Treatment of each case depends on the diagnosis and whether the vet can physically solve the problem.

- **Resolution of torsion via the vagina**

  This involves rotating both the foetus and the uterine horn in which it is located. The veterinary surgeon should always work in the opposite direction to the torsion, i.e. in the case of anti-clockwise torsion (viewed from the rear), the foetus should be rotated clockwise.

  It is preferable not to rupture the allantoic or amniotic bags, although in many cases this is impossible to avoid.

  - **If the presentation of the foetus is longitudinal and cephalic,** the vet must rotate the calf while supporting the nape of its neck. This manoeuvre requires strength and skill. It may also help to secure the jaw of the calf with a rope to pull the head towards the entrance of the cervix. It may also help to

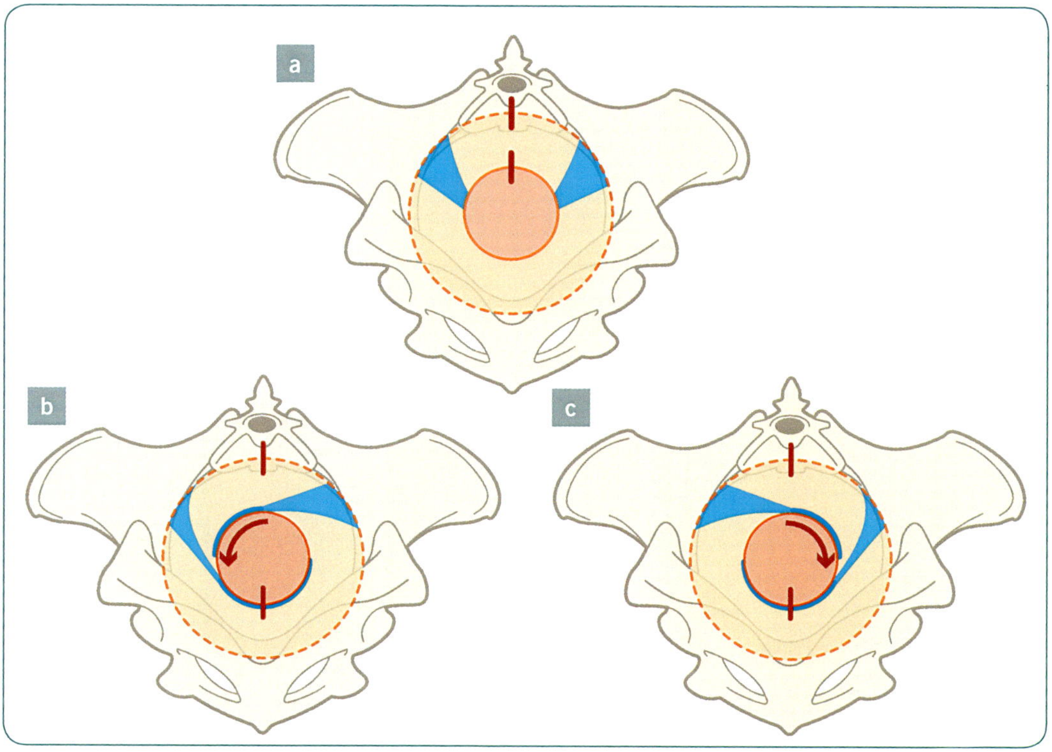

Figure 17. Schematic drawing showing a normal uterus (a), left uterine torsion (b) and uterine torsion (c).

externalise one of the forelimbs, although in other cases the limbs must be forced backwards and bent so that pressure can be applied to the calf's head. Another useful approach is to apply upwards pressure on the outside of the abdomen using a plank, or alternatively to have two people squat (one on each side) and support the cow's abdomen with their backs. No two uterine torsions are the same, and the approaches used for successful resolution can vary widely. Traction should be maintained until the spinal column of the calf passes the linea alba of the mother, at which point the tension diminishes.

After correcting the torsion, the vet must assist the calving cow. Depending on the degree of dilation of the cow, the calf should be extracted (by first facilitating dilation of the cervix), or physiological dilation should be allowed to progress and the situation should be reviewed after two hours. Calving normally proceeds smoothly after resolution of torsion, unless there is another cause of dystocia. In cases of uterine torsion, the calf requires immediate attention upon delivery to clear the airways.

It is important to monitor the elasticity of the cervix, which can easily rupture. Hasty extraction of the foetus can trigger uterine prolapse.

- **If the foetus presents in the posterior position,** the veterinary surgeon should hold the buttocks of the calf and attempt to rotate it. Often, it is necessary to tie the lowermost hindlimb to prevent the calf from moving towards the abdomen when applying rotational force. The extraction process should be approached with even more care than in cases of anterior presentation, as both dilation and extraction are more complicated when the foetus presents in the posterior position.
- **Rolling technique**

  If the veterinary surgeon cannot correct the position of the calf via the vagina, he/she may have to resort to rolling the mother. This solution can be adopted from the outset. The rolling method involves immobilising some part of the foetus (legs, head, or both) and rolling the cow so that it rotates around the uterus, which remains fixed and immobile due to traction exerted upon the foetus from the outside (Fig. 18).

  When the direction of the torsion has been determined (as viewed from the rear), the cow should be carefully cast on the side on which the torsion is located. For example, if the direction of the torsion is anti-clockwise, the cow should be cast on its left side in a spacious area with good bedding. The forelimbs and hindlimbs are bound in such a way that no pressure is exerted on the abdomen, and a rope is attached to the calf. Next, the cow is rolled towards the side on which the torsion is located and the outcome assessed by vaginal or rectal examination. If the procedure is not successful, the cow should be rolled again, and the torsion re-evaluated. The postpartum care required in these cases is the same as for other cases of dystocia.
- **Caesarean section**

  If the torsion cannot be manually corrected or if another dystocia subsequently arises that cannot be resolved (insufficient dilation, foetal disproportion), a caesarean section should be performed.

  When conducting a caesarean section to resolve a uterine torsion, in addition to the standard surgical precautions, it is essential that the uterus be handled with extreme care. The pressures to which this organ is subjected make it a very fragile structure. It is advisable to support the uterus at several points when attempting to resolve uterine torsion. It is not recommended to use the fingers, as the uterus may tear; instead, use the back of the hand, the fist or the forearm. After correcting the position of the uterus, the vet can proceed with the surgery and should ultimately thoroughly examine the uterus and the suture.

Maternal diseases

Maternal diseases can directly or indirectly cause dystocia.

Hypocalcaemia

While clinical hypocalcaemia can appear before calving, subclinical hypocalcaemia can be already present in the early stages of labour.

As calcium is directly involved in uterine contractions, hypocalcaemia can induce uterine inertia in the cow. Moreover, depending on the degree of hypocalcaemia, the cow may have difficulty rising. In the early stages of labour, the mother will often repeatedly stand up and lie back down in order to appropriately position the calf for calving.

Mastitis

During the preparation phase, the presence of mastitis, whether clinical or subclinical, can significantly influence calving. Immunosuppression, oedema and inflammation of the mammary gland at the time of delivery, as well as inadequate handling or housing, can result in acute mastitis (with or without toxaemia), which affects the progression of calving. Mastitis can influence certain stages of labour or result in retention of the placenta. In cases of mastitis with septicaemia, calving is usually premature and the calf may not survive. On the

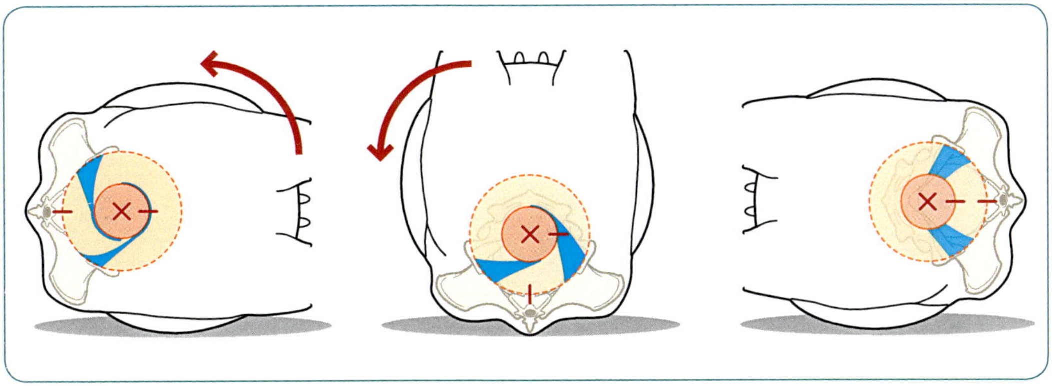

Figure 18. Schematic showing the resolution of an anticlockwise torsion by rolling the cow.

other hand, cows with mastitis with toxaemia are themselves unlikely to survive (Fig. 19).

Lameness

Lameness in cows should be addressed as soon as possible, as lame animals will not feed properly, their body condition will deteriorate and they will be less well prepared to deal with the immunosuppression that accompanies pregnancy. Moreover, depending on the type of lameness, the cow may adopt abnormal postures, which in turn can promote the development of other diseases (e.g. LDA, RDA, joint problems, pressure sores). Thus, it is generally only a matter of time before dystocia occurs in lame pregnant cows.

It is important to try to resolve lameness in cows as soon as possible.

Fat cow syndrome

Fat cow syndrome may be caused by reproductive failure or by poor handling. The excess body condition typical of this syndrome is usually observed in dry cows, as these cows show significant alterations in their reproductive rates (increased postpartum intervals, long dry periods, or both). Females with fat cow syndrome undergo significant alterations in metabolism, have functionally impaired, fatty livers, and can suffer other disorders such as ketosis and hypocalcaemia. In many cases, these cows also develop "downer cow syndrome" (see Case 6, p. 126).

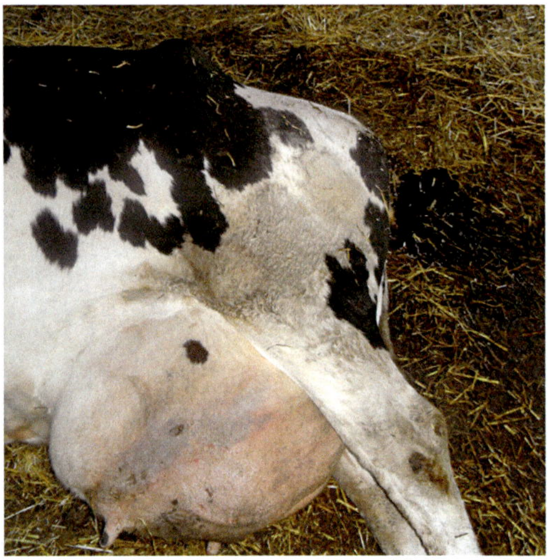

Figure 19. A cow in the final days of gestation that has succumbed to mastitis with toxaemia. Symptoms of this disease include lateral prostration, cyanosis of the udder and bloody diarrhoea.

Changes in environment (facilities and handling) as causes of dystocia

For a pregnancy to properly come to term, it is important to avoid sudden changes in the cow's environment and to carefully monitor the female just before calving. It is also essential that the personnel assisting the calving are sufficiently capable and qualified to deliver the calf:

- It is important to monitor the health of the female during pregnancy and calving (trips to the feeder, body condition, temperature, rumen fill, manure quality, udder health, etc.).

- Avoid changes in the cow's housing and batch, and in the personnel that handle the animal.
- Affected cows are easily stressed and should not be subjected to aggressive manipulations (no shouting, or striking).
- Designated calving areas should be properly equipped, clean and well ventilated, comfortable, with clean drinking water and non-slip floors. Moreover, they should be easy to access and allow unintrusive monitoring of calving cows.
- It is crucial that all materials required for calving and postpartum care are clean and ready.
- It is important to be patient, but also to know when to intervene in the event that calving does not proceed as normal. In cases of postural dystocia, uterine torsion or the concurrent conditions described above, it is important to act quickly.

When to suspect and how to confirm dystocia

When it is clear that calving has begun, the cow should be more closely monitored, without interfering with the calving process. It is important to monitor:

- **Dilation of the teat cistern.** Cows usually calve 6-12 hours after the dilation of teat cistern.
- **Milk ejection.** A cow can eject milk for several reasons unrelated to calving, such as compressive oedema (common in heifers) or stress induced by various causes. Milk ejection occurs during the expulsion phase of labour, when the cow is ready to calve, but may also be observed in cases of uterine torsion and other dystocias (Fig. 16).

HOW TO DETECT DYSTOCIA

To confirm dystocia, it is essential to review all the animal's data: age, calving number, days of gestation, breed of cow and bull, previous diseases, etc. A careful vaginal examination should also be performed and the findings confirmed by rectal examination. The following questions should be answered:

1. Has the cervix been palpated? Is uterine torsion suspected?
2. Is the cervix partially or fully dilated?
3. Are any unusual odours detected?
4. Can the allantoic sac be touched in the area between the cervix and vagina?
5. Has the allantoic sac ruptured? Have any prior examinations been performed?
6. Is the foetus malpresented?
7. Can more than one foetus be felt (i.e. more than two legs or one head)?
8. Are there any signs of placenta praevia?
9. Can you identify what you are touching?
10. Does the cow appear to have any disease at the time of calving?

- **If the cow does not lie down or repeatedly stands up.** This may indicate discomfort and restlessness. When the typical signs of calving are observed but the cow does not lie down, even when in comfortable surroundings, this usually suggests dystocia (due to a disproportionate foetus or malpresentation), which bothers the cow when lying down. Possible signs of colic (striking the abdominal area with the head or one of the legs) should also be assessed.

Box 1. Diagnostic algorithm for calving when cervix is closed: vaginal examination.

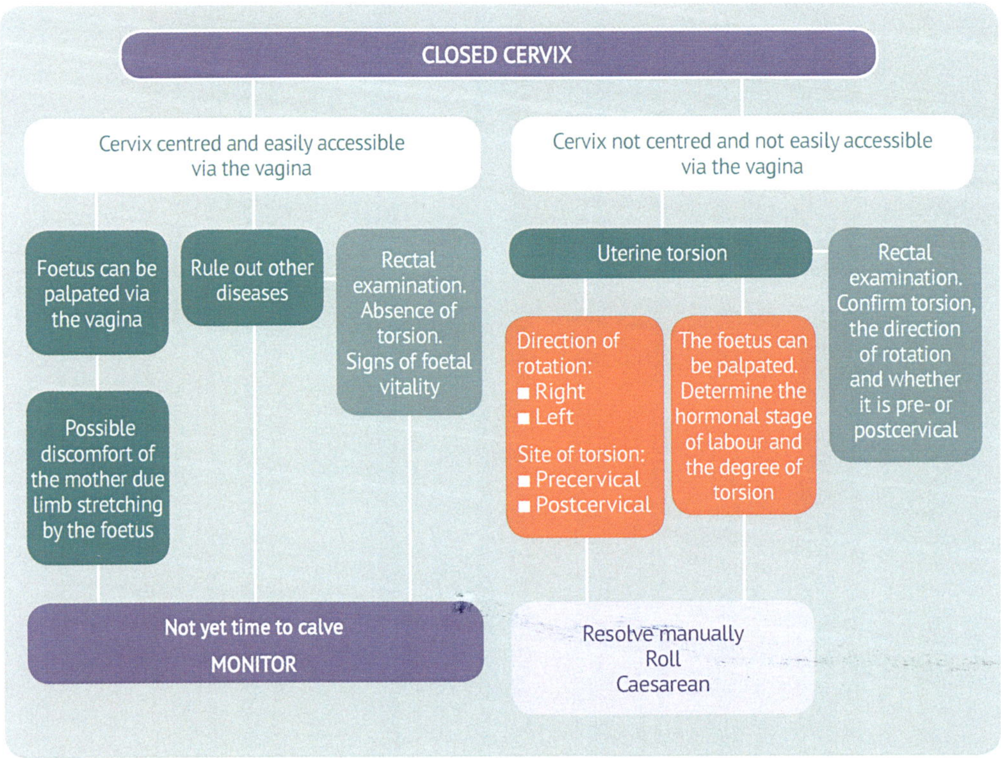

Box2. Diagnostic algorithm for calving when cervix is open: vaginal examination.

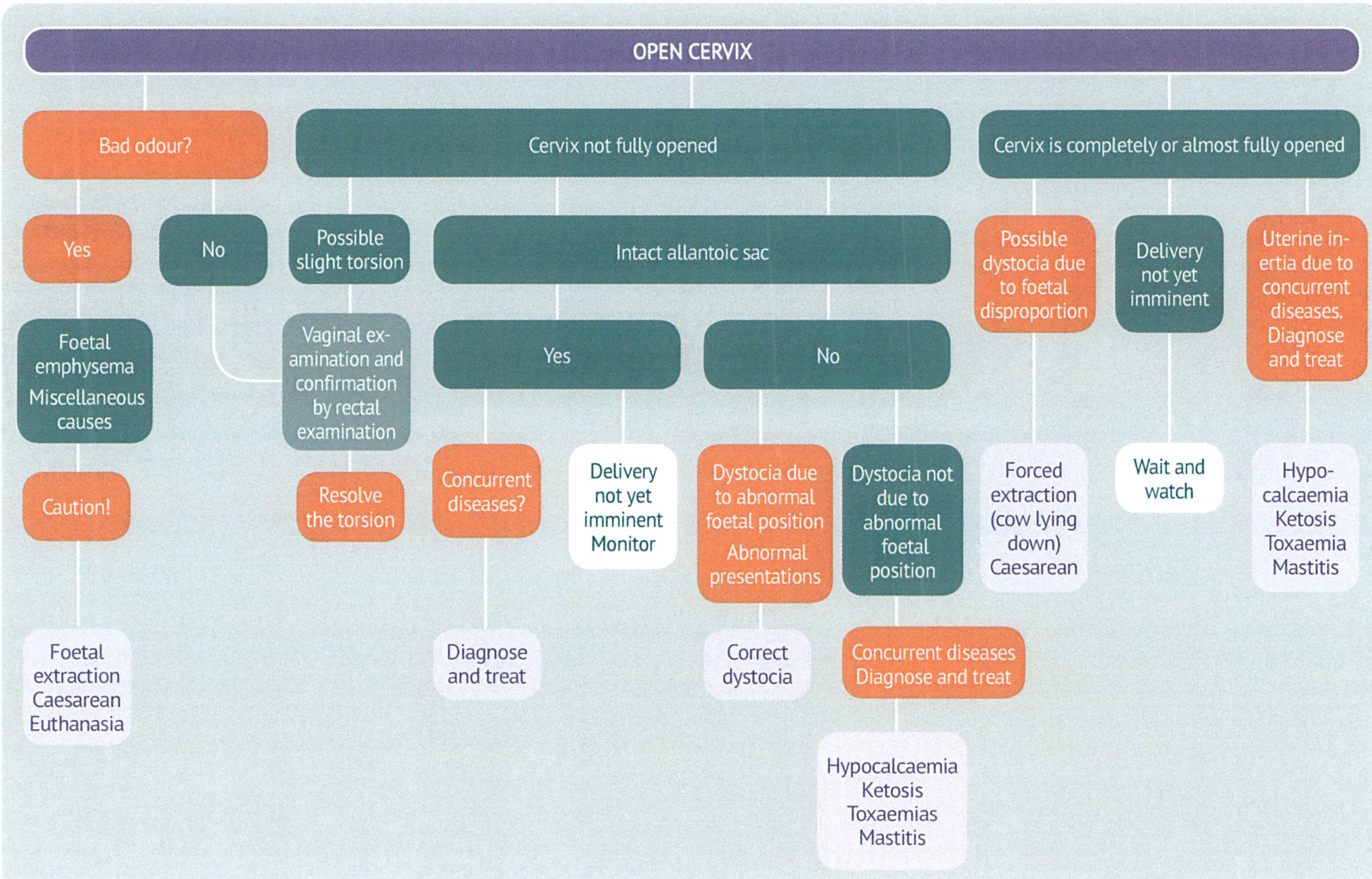

4

Nutrition and body condition

Diet management

Managing the cow's diet during the peripartum period is crucial to ensure maximum milk production. During this period, the cow should be thought of as a "luxury item", and treated accordingly. Unfortunately, this is not always the case. Diet management has been discussed in many scientific publications, and a wide range of different strategies proposed.

The peripartum cow can be compared to an aircraft that has reached its destination, and must now prepare for its next flight. Thus, dairy cows go through the following stages:

- Touchdown: the cow is dried off and stops producing milk (dry period).
- Maintenance: the dry period.
- Taxiing and take-off: the cow prepares to calve and to produce milk once again.

Obviously, bringing a cow that produces 28 litres of milk per day to zero litres during the dry period and back up to a lactation peak of over 60 litres, all the while maintaining adequate body condition, will differ to drying off a cow that produces only 10 litres and preparing her to reach a peak of 30 litres of milk per day.

Case studies on dry cow management

Case 1

This animal is a high-yield cow. Figures 1, 2 and 3 show the official milk production data obtained from two milkings over three lactations (www.cowsulting.com).

- As shown in Figure 1, the cow ends lactation with values of 29-30 litres of milk and over 400 days in milk. The cow then calves and reaches a peak of about 72 litres at week 14 of lactation.
- Figure 2 shows the lactation curve of the cow. As seen in Figure 3, production levels are well above the average for any group of cattle on the farm.

Case 2

This case concerns a medium yielding cow. Figure 4 shows the official milk production data obtained for two milkings over two lactations (www.cowsulting.com).

- As shown in Figure 4, the cow ends the lactation period with approximately 18 litres of milk and just under 400 days in milk, peaking at 38 litres around week nine of lactation.

Figure 1. Milk production for Case 1. Data are presented as a point cloud representing litres of milk collected as a function of days in milk (over all lactations).

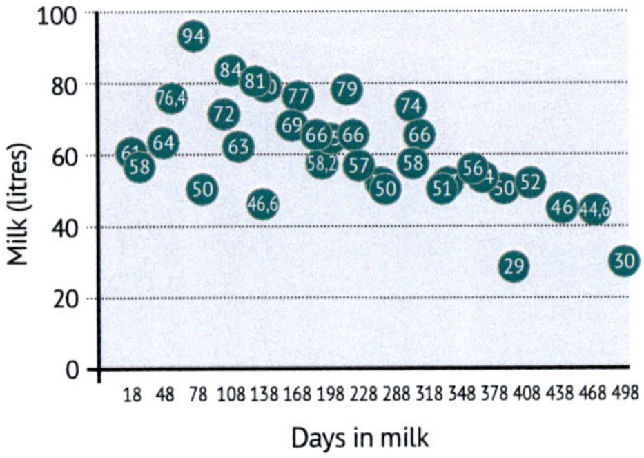

Figure 2. Lactation curve based on milk production data for the cow in Case 1. Wood method. Source: www.cowsulting.com.

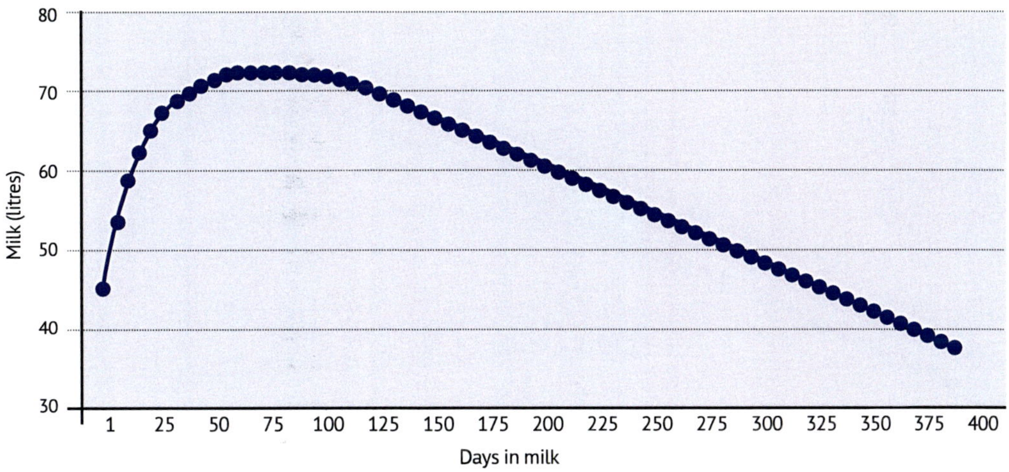

Figure 3. Lactation curve for cow in Case 1 compared with the mean lactation curves for the same farm for three different lactations. Wood method. Source: www.cowsulting.com.

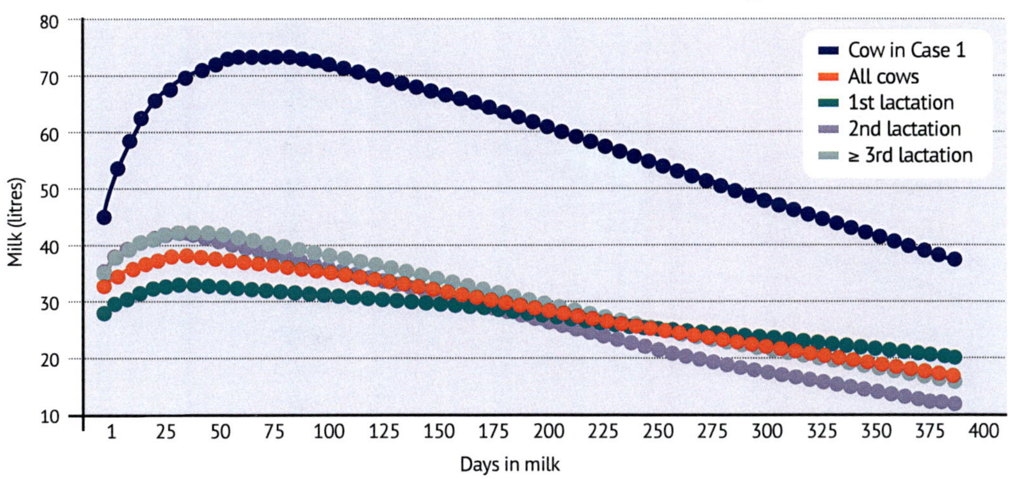

Case 3

This case concerns a low-yield cow. Figure 5 shows the official milk production data for two milkings over three lactations (www.cowsulting.com).

- As shown in Figure 5, the cow ends its lactation with less than 14 litres of milk and under 400 days in milk, peaking at 24 litres in week 13 of lactation.

The cows featured in each of the three cases come from the same farm, which has an average production of 33.5 litres of milk per day and a mean peak of 38 litres at week nine of lactation.

Figure 4. Milk production data for cow in Case 2. Data are presented as a point cloud representing the litres of milk collected as a function of the days in milk of the cow. Source: www.cowsulting.com.

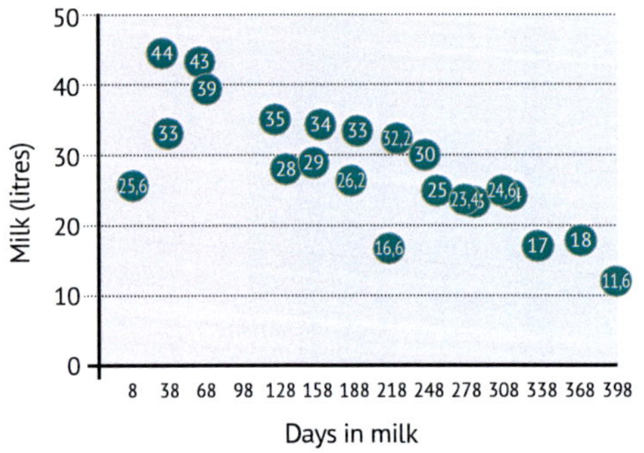

Figure 5. Lactation curve based on milk production data for cow in Case 2. Wood method. Source: www.cowsulting.com.

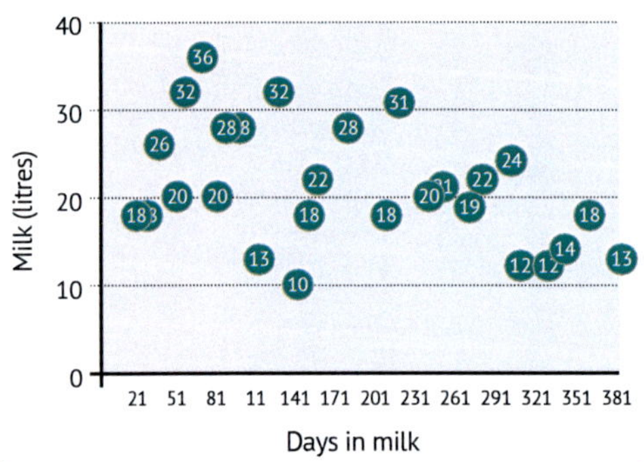

Given that the standard deviation of the farm is estimated at 9.49 litres, rations should be calculated for a single batch based on a production of 43 litres (mean production + standard deviation) in order not to penalise high-yield cows (Case 1).

However, drawbacks of this approach include squandering feed and fattening less productive cows (Case 3).

While scientists have proposed different strategies to address this problem, it should be borne in mind that it is not always possible to extrapolate experimental scenarios to real cases, including those described here. In general, scientists tend to study more extreme scenarios, which are more difficult to deal with on an actual farm.

A cow that initially consumes a corn silage ration of 35 kg/day containing 27 % starch, and that is subsequently given another ration of hay and pasture during the dry period to promote increased consumption of feed and corn silage, will undergo a more physiologically aggressive change than one on a ration of 22 kg corn silage per day containing 22 % starch. In our opinion, the ideal scenario is that the starting point and endpoint be as similar as possible.

Regardless of the number of days required for the rumen flora of the cow to adapt to the aforementioned changes, the less aggressive the changes in diet, the better the overall health of the cow.

It is imperative that the cow begins and ends the peripartum period in the best condition possible.

If these conditions are fulfilled, the cow's appetite will increase progressively, which is the best possible result. It is widely agreed that postpartum diseases generally occur because the cow has not fully recovered from the negative energy balance of the postpartum period. It is thus important to aim for a phased and gradual increase in the cow's intake capacity (Fig. 6), and to provide them with palatable feed that stimulates intake.

Figure 6. Dry matter intake around the time of calving (Bell, 1997).

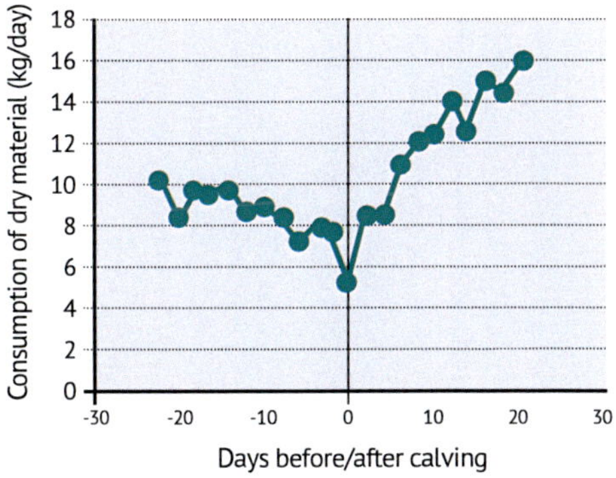

The importance of diet

Consider the following practical example: imagine that a farmer carefully follows all the appropriate recommendations to ensure that a cow reaches the moment of calving in good health. The cow successfully recuperates, but is subsequently fed with winter silage (Fig. 7) that has not accumulated enough sugar content due to low levels of sunlight. Moreover, the silage has an unpleasant odour due to the accumulation of butyric acid, which forms due to a lack of sufficient sugar sources (e.g. beet pulp, corn grain, preservatives) required to improve fermentation. This results in unwanted fermentation of the silage. Consequently, the cow does not consume the quantities necessary to offset its negative energy balance, triggering a cascade of metabolic problems and a significant change in its condition.

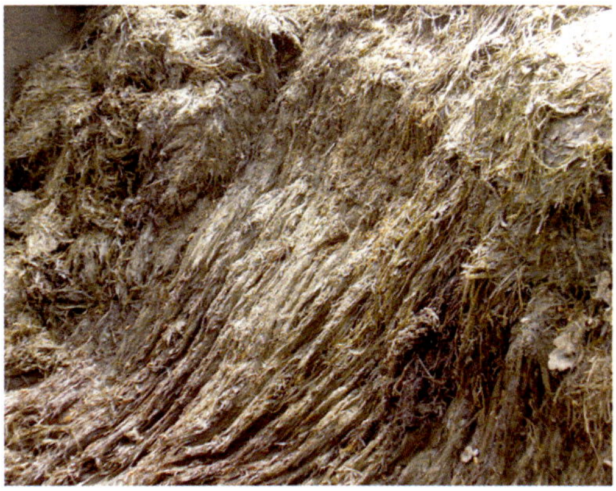

Figure 7. Poorly maintained winter silage (extreme case). This type of silage should never be given to dairy cattle.

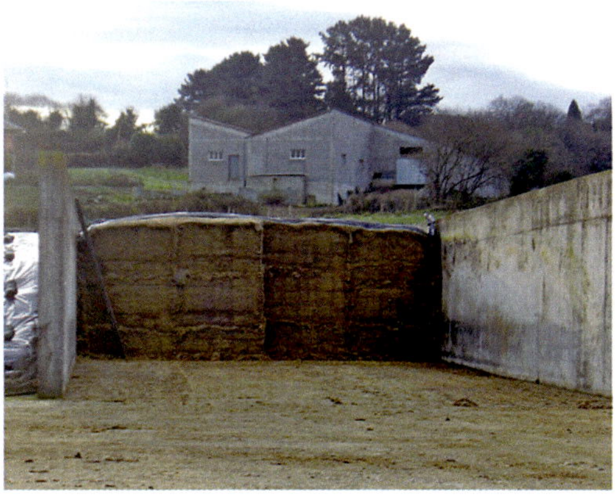

Figure 8. Good-quality silos are required. Silage should be removed from the silo in portions corresponding to the number of cows to be fed (0.15 m/day in summer; 0.10 m/day in winter).

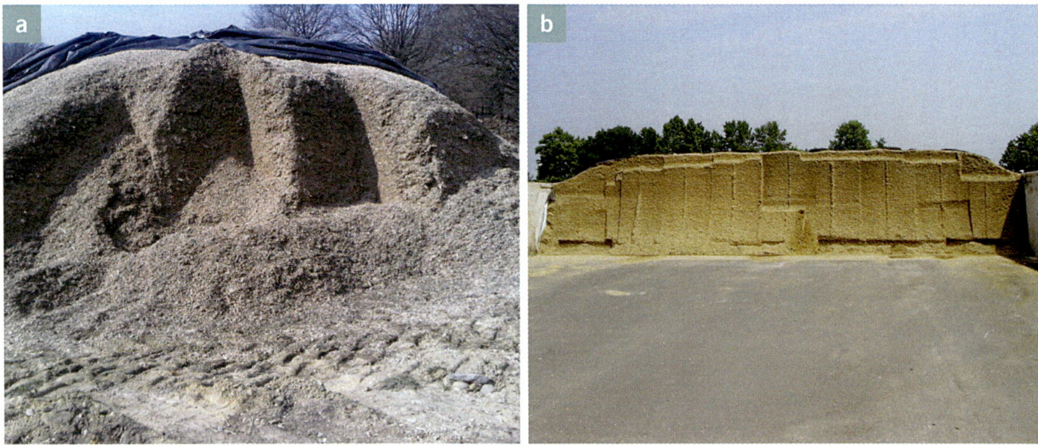

Figure 9. The manner in which the forage is removed affects its subsequent preservation in the silo. The forage in silo (a) will not be preserved as well as that in silo (b).

When poorly preserved, fungi, yeast or fungal toxins can grow in silage (Figs. 10, 11 and 12). Consumption of contaminated silage can trigger a range of diseases with different clinical symptoms. Postpartum cows that are fed contaminated silage can develop immunosuppressive conditions, which can in turn lead to mastitis, lameness, indigestion, etc. Silage contaminated with these types of pathogens can also impair rumination and cause appetite loss, dysbiosis, bloating and diarrhoea.

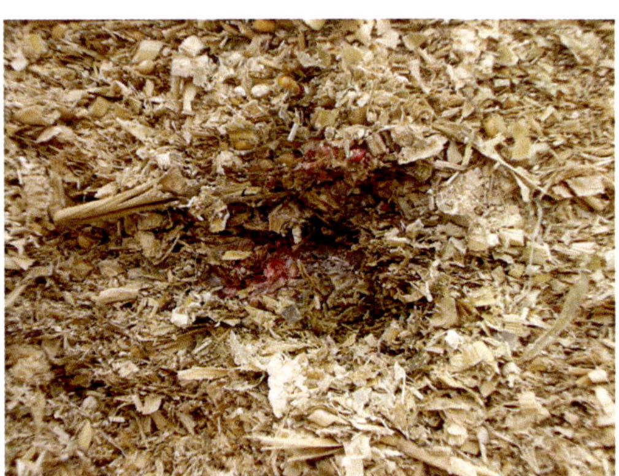

Figure 10. Corn silage containing red fungi (*Fusarium, Monascus*).

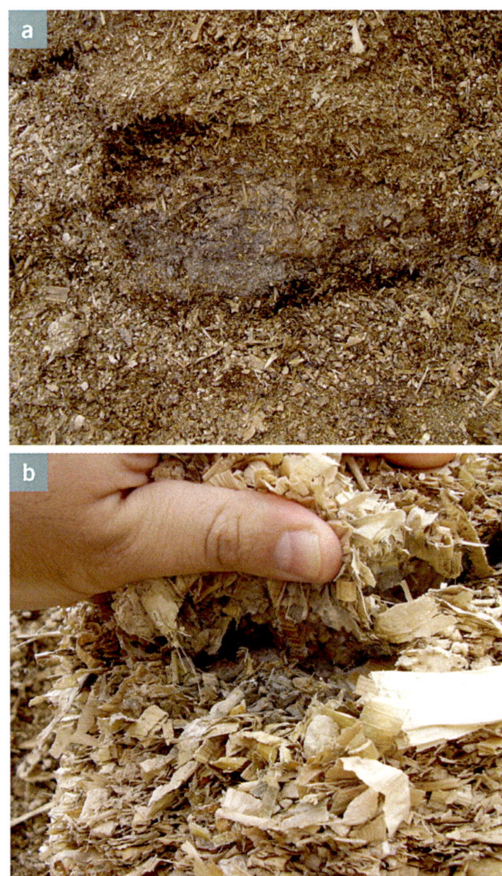

Figure 11. Corn silage containing white fungi (*Geotrichum, Byssochlamys*; order *Mucorales*).

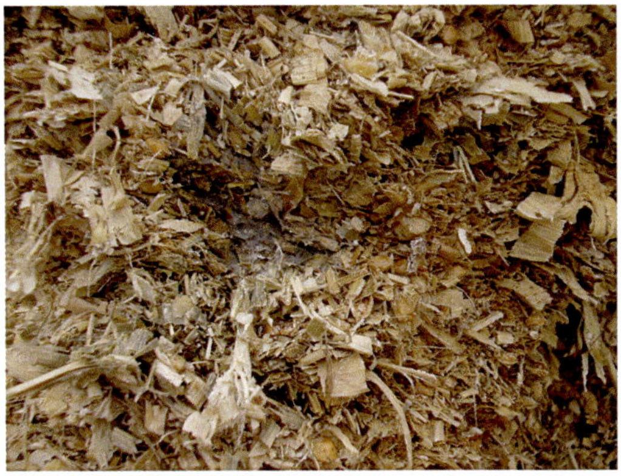

Figure 12. Corn silage containing white to greenish-blue fungus (*Penicillium*). This fungus has the highest toxic potential due to its neurotoxic effects.

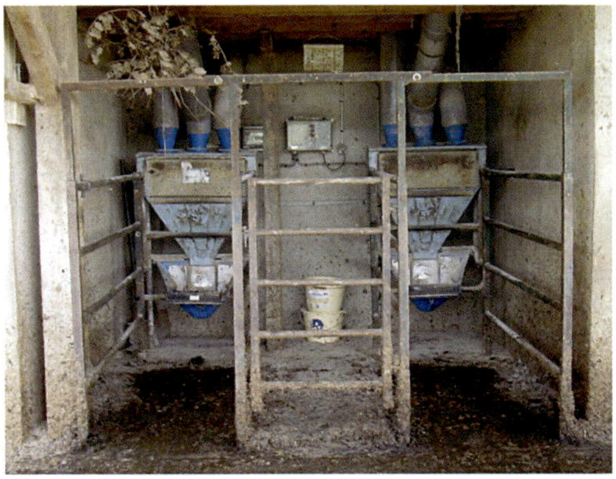

Figure 13. The ACD system allows individualised dosing of specific feed types. Note the three downspouts for two concentrates and the corrector spout.

Food distribution methods

Automatic concentrate distribution (ACD)

The automatic concentrate distribution (ACD) system uses individual collar devices that identify each cow and thus allows progressive regulation of the amount of feed provided (Fig. 13). For example, this method allows reduction of the ration from 8 to 0 kg of concentrate over 10 days in preparation for drying-off and an increase from 0 to 6 kg (or 1 % of body weight) over a period of 15 days prior to calving (or 25 days in the case of heifers). Using this method, the cow can be "challenged" after calving with increasing amounts of feed, not exceeding 0.5 kg/cow/day, until peak lactation is reached. This is the perfect tool to provide each individual cow with the necessary dietary requirements and to avoid both excesses and deficits in the diet.

Unifeed system

Using the Unifeed system for a single batch of high-yield cows, rations are generated for a specific animal type, and thus individualisation is not possible. Usually the mean ration for the farm plus one standard deviation is taken as a reference.

The result obtained using this method largely depends on how closely the requirements of a given cow correspond to the mean ration of the farm. This is influenced by genetic quality, reproductive imbalances and pathological processes in the herd (even when cows are genetically very similar).

Rations can be individualised to some extent when using the Unifeed system to feed prepartum batches and high or low-yield cows. However, this system can only be used on farms of a certain minimum size. Changes to a different batch should be carefully controlled in order to minimise stress.

Diet and production

To ensure that cattle are well fed, a variety of feed additives can be used. While these can help to mitigate dietary shortcomings in many cases, they will not eradicate underlying problems. For example, anionic salts can be added to alleviate subclinical hypocalcaemia. However, the veterinary surgeon should always focus on the underlying problems that cause these diseases.

PROCEDURES TO CONTROL RATION PRODUCTIVITY

- Ration control.
- Control of body condition.
- Control of the lactation curve.

Lactation curve

If the relevant protocols and appropriate recommendations are followed during the dry period and early lactation, the cow will reach peak lactation at the right time. One should aim for a good quantity of milk at peak lactation; one litre extra at peak lactation translates to about 200 litres over the remainder of the lactation period.

Ideal lactation curves for both primiparous and multiparous cows are shown in Table 1 and Figures 14 and 15. The time point at which peak lactation should be reached, according to INRA (2007), is also shown. These examples can be used as references and compared with the actual lactation curve of a farm or a specific cow. It is always preferable to analyse data derived from automated milking systems, which take daily measurements that are corrected according to whether milking occurs in the morning or afternoon. In the absence of this type of system, a lactation curve can be generated using the lactation record. Wood's gamma function can be used to evaluate the collected data.

Cows are thinnest approximately 15 days prior to peak lactation. This information is crucial to understand the progression of lactation and to determine:

1. If there has been any failure in the management of the peripartum period, due to:
   - not achieving the appropriate increase in dry matter intake.
   - the cow not recovering from the negative energy balance.
   - not providing the cow with a sufficiently palatable ration containing the appropriate energy and protein density.
2. If fertility is diminished. The sooner a cow exits the period of negative energy balance, which usually happens after peak lactation, the greater the probability that it can become pregnant again. However, the more this transition is delayed, the longer it will take the cow to become pregnant again.

Case studies on peak lactation

Case 1

Farm with lactation peak at five weeks in adult cows and at nine weeks in first-calf heifers, in line with the ideal scenario shown in Table 2. Improved fertility is observed from peak lactation onwards.

Case 2

Farm with peak lactation at week eight of lactation in adult cows and week fifteen in first-calf heifers (Table 3). The peak lactation value is lower than that seen in Case 1, and thus fertility is reduced comparatively.

Table 1. Milk production potential (kg/day) of a lactating cow as a function of calving number, the total production potential at 305 days of lactation, and the production potential at peak lactation (successful insemination on day 90 of lactation) (INRA 2007).

Primiparous cows (heifers)	Milk production potential for 305 days of lactation (kg)							
Week of lactation	4,000	5,000	6,000	7,000	8,000	9,000	10,000	11,000
	Milk production (kg/day)							
1	11	14	17	19	22	25	28	30
2	13	16	19	23	26	29	32	35
3	14	18	21	25	28	32	35	39
4	15	19	23	26	30	34	38	41
8	16	20	24	28	32	35	39	43
12	15	19	23	27	31	34	38	42
16	15	18	22	26	29	33	37	40
20	14	18	21	25	28	32	35	39
24	14	17	20	24	27	30	34	37
28	13	16	19	23	26	29	32	35
32	12	15	18	22	25	28	31	34
36	12	15	17	20	23	26	29	32
40	11	14	16	19	22	24	27	30
44	10	12	14	17	19	22	24	26
Multiparous cows (adults)	**Milk production potential for 305 days of lactation (kg)**							
Week of lactation	5,000	6,000	7,000	8,000	9,000	10,000	11,000	12,000
	Milk production (kg/day)							
1	19	22	26	30	34	37	41	45
2	21	25	30	34	38	42	46	51
3	22	27	31	36	40	45	49	53
4	23	27	32	36	41	45	50	54
8	22	26	30	35	39	43	48	52
12	20	24	28	32	36	40	44	49
16	19	23	26	30	34	38	41	45
20	18	21	25	28	32	35	39	42
24	16	20	23	26	29	33	36	39
28	15	18	21	24	27	30	33	36
32	14	17	20	22	25	28	31	34
36	13	15	18	20	23	25	28	30
40	11	13	16	18	20	22	24	27
44	9	11	12	14	16	18	19	21

Figure 14. Ideal lactation curve for primiparous cows (INRA 2007).

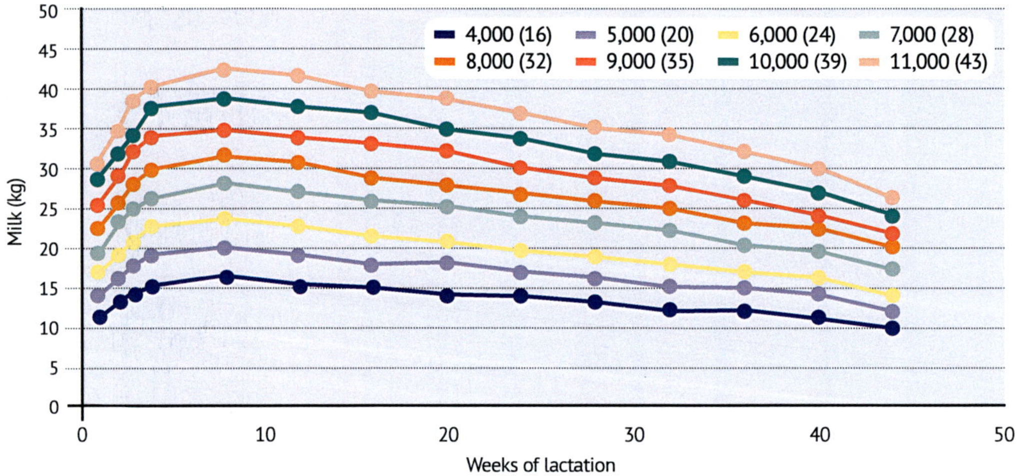

Figure 15. Ideal lactation curve for multiparous cows (adult) (INRA 2007).

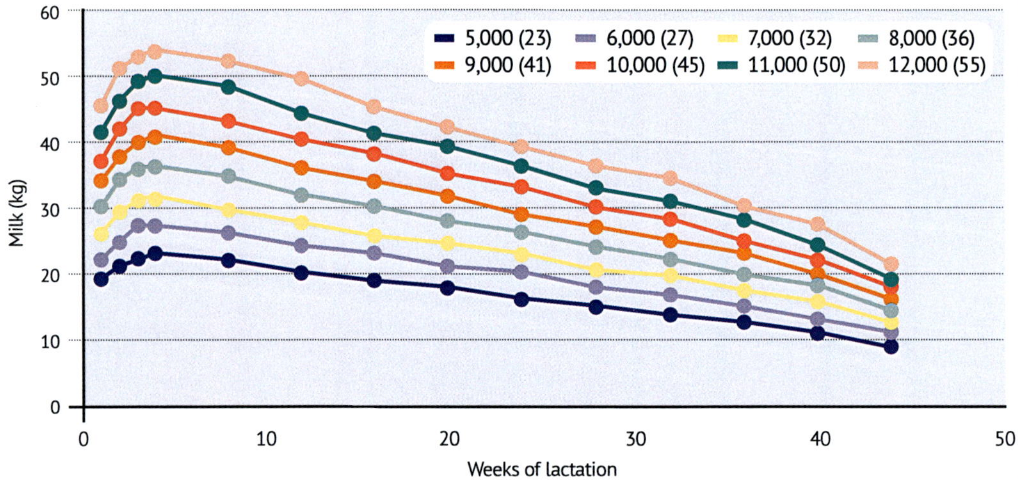

Table 2. Compiled milk production data for farm in Case 1. Source: www.cowsulting.com.

Lactations	Total production (daily production)	Peak lactation (week)	Lactation persistence (weekly-monthly decrease)
All	9,679 (31.73 l/day)	38.52 (6)	98.39 % (1.61 % - 6.44 %)
1st calf	8,175 (26.8 l/day)	30.62 (9)	98.74 % (1.26 % - 5.04 %)
2nd calf	9,695 (31.79 l/day)	41.16 (6)	97.85 % (2.15 % - 8.6 %)
≥ 3rd calf	10,528 (34.52 l/day)	42.96 (5)	98.33 % (1.67 % - 6.68 %)

Table 3. Compiled milk production data for dairy farm in Case 2.
Source: www.cowsulting.com.

Lactations	Total production (daily production)	Peak lactation (week)	Lactation persistence (weekly-monthly decrease)
All	9,991 (32.76 l/day)	35.56 (10)	99.19 % (0.81 % - 3.24 %)
1st calf	9,097 (29.83 l/day)	31.17 (15)	99.5 % (0.5 % - 2 %)
2nd calf	10,833 (35.52 l/day)	39.84 (6)	99.08 % (0.92 % - 3.68 %)
≥ 3rd calf	10,770 (35.31 l/day)	41.21 (8)	98.6 % (1.4 % - 5.6 %)

The big difference between the farms in Cases 1 and 2 is that while the former uses a grazing system, feeds the cows grass silage and distributes approximately 9 kg of concentrate per cow per day using the ACD system, the second farm maximises the use of fodder, administering only 6.5 kg of concentrate per cow per day using the Unifeed system to produce a single ration. The second farm obtains good yields (33 litres/cow/day with 198 g concentrate/litre milk) and high intakes of 22.5 kg dry matter/cow/day, using rations with not particularly high energy densities (0.94 UFL/kg dry matter). In this scenario, fresh cows, which require high energy and protein densities due to their lower intake, are at a disadvantage. Therefore, despite the good results achieved in Case 2, it would be preferable to individualise the rations of cows that are within the first three months postpartum.

Table 4. Compiled milk production data for farm in Case 3.
Source: www.cowsulting.com.

Months of lactation	Number of cows	Milk (l)	Days in lactation
1	5	26.52	12.8
2	5	25.16	45
3	2	22	77
4	2	17.1	116.5
5	4	22.95	139.5
6	2	12.9	159
7	3	19	191.33
8	7	20.57	218.57
9	6	17.27	263.33
≥ 10	5	17.32	312.6
Media	41	20.62	165.83

Case 3

Dairy farm in which cows are not reaching appropriate mean productivity in the first 90 days of lactation (Table 4) (Fig. 16). This farm has low yields in all months of lactation.

Given that the farm in Case 3 uses the Unifeed system to produce a single ration, the only way to increase the yield is to calculate the ration based on a higher milk production value (i.e. increase the ration).

How to predict and improve production potential

Several simple rules can be used to estimate the production potential of a cow at peak lactation. The INRA 2007 proposes the following formula:

Figure 16. Lactation curves for the herd in Case 2 obtained from data from milk records. Wood method. Source: www.cowsulting.com.

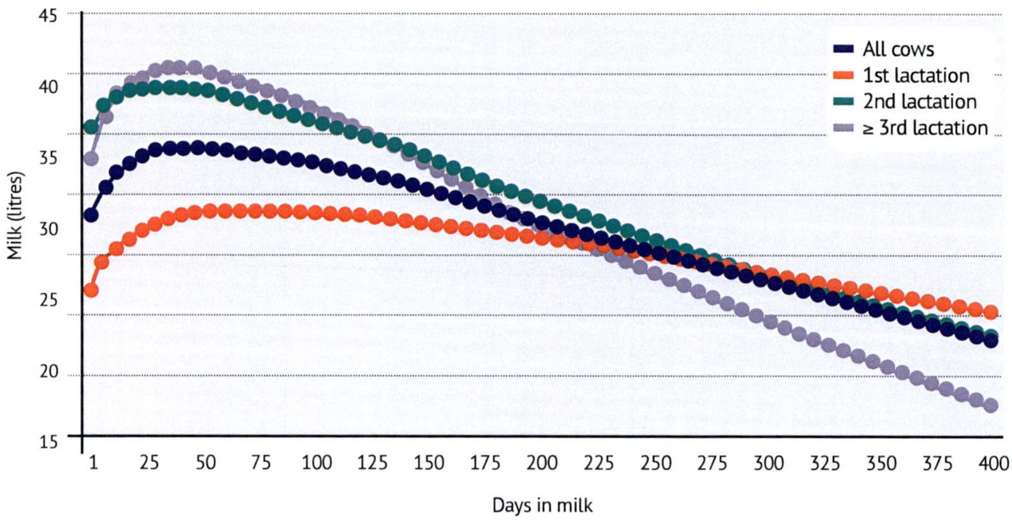

$$P_{max\ pot} = ((P_4+P_5+P_6)/3) \times 0.84 + 13$$

$P_{max\ pot}$: maximum milk production (potential)

P: milk production

- The maximum milk production (potential) is equal to the mean production on days 4, 5 and 6 multiplied by 0.84, plus 13.
- To calculate the milk production potential at 305 days using this equation, multiply by 224 (in the case of multiparous cows) or 259 (for primiparous cows) (INRA 2007).

Predicting the milk potential of a cow permits the calculation of the amount of concentrate with which the cow will be "challenged". As a general rule, cows should be exhaustively monitored during the first week postpartum, and for longer if any problems are detected. This extra monitoring is a worthwhile investment, as it can ultimately bring in additional revenue.

IMPROVING MILK POTENTIAL

- On farms that do not use an automatic concentrate dispenser, one convenient way to control feeding is to supplement the Unifeed ration with a balanced and palatable feed for at least 10 days. Accordingly, cows that do not increase their feed intake after calving can be easily identified. It is also advisable to record the yield in the milk parlour on postpartum days 4, 5 and 6.
- If a farm has a low-yield production batch, fresh cows can be incorporated into this batch for one week so that they adapt their intake before being transferred to the high-yield batch.

Body condition

Measurement of the body condition score (BCS) is a necessary and useful means of monitoring the state of the herd (Table 5). While there are many recommendations on assessing body condition, we recommend evaluating the ischium, ileum, scapula, back and ribs, and scoring the animal on a scale of 0 to 5 (Fig. 17).

While determining the body condition score is somewhat subjective, this is not problematic as long as the animals are always scored by the same person (Fig. 18). However, if animals are scored by more than one person, it is important that there are no differences greater than 0.5 points between observers to ensure that no changes in category occur (e.g. a change from 2.5 to 3 points). To account for potential differences, scoring can be performed in increments of 0.25 points.

The evaluation of body condition can be made a monthly routine (e.g. when cows are immobilised for reproductive examination) and can provide important information. It may be useful to also score locomotion; this way the state of the legs and hocks, which also influence production, can be assessed. The software used on each farm evaluates the data entered and determines the mean values, which are then used as references for the herd.

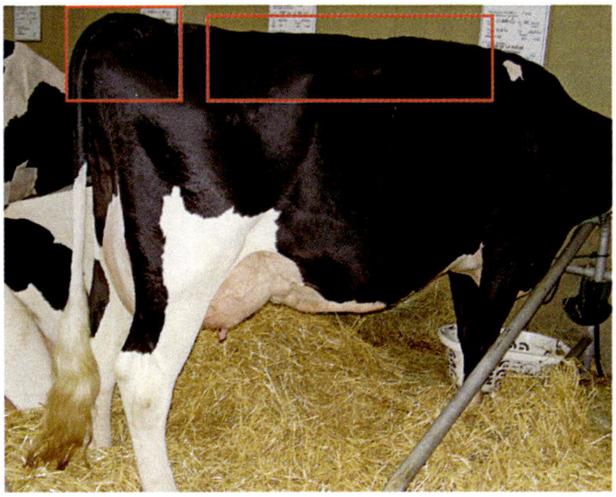

Figure 17. Assessment of body condition.

Case studies on body condition

Case 1

This farm has 40 cows that are fed using the Unifeed system. In general, the cows have BCS values that fit well with the ideal curve shown in Fig. 19.

Table 5. Recommended body condition score based on lactation status.

Stage of lactation	Days in milk	Body condition score		
		Objective (BCS)	Min.	Max.
Calving	0	3.50	3.25	3.75
Early lactation	1 to 30	3.00	2.75	3.25
Peak lactation	31 to 100	2.75	2.50	3.00
Mid lactation	101 to 200	3.00	2.75	3.25
Late lactation	201 to 300	3.25	3.00	3.75
Drying-off	> 300	3.50	3.25	3.75
Dry period	- 60 to -1	3.50	3.25	3.75

Figure 18. Graphical representation of ideal body condition scores. Source: www.cowsulting.com.

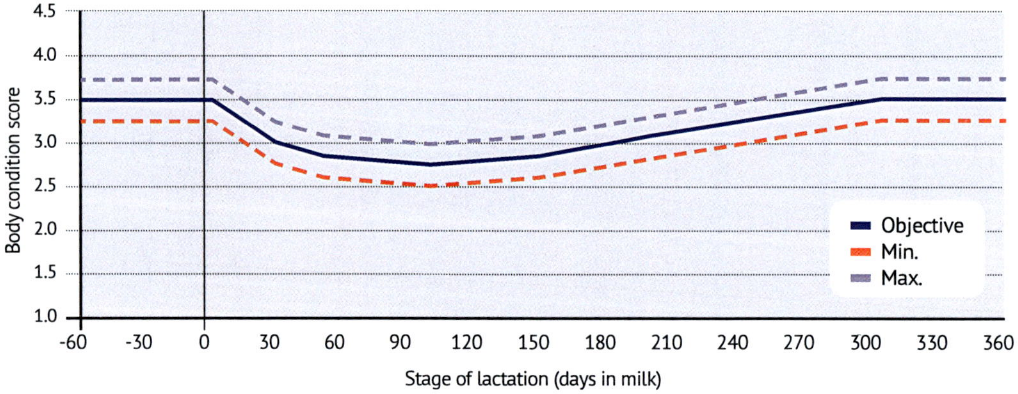

Figure 19. Graphical representation of body condition scores in Case 1 as compared with recommended values. Source: www.cowsulting.com.

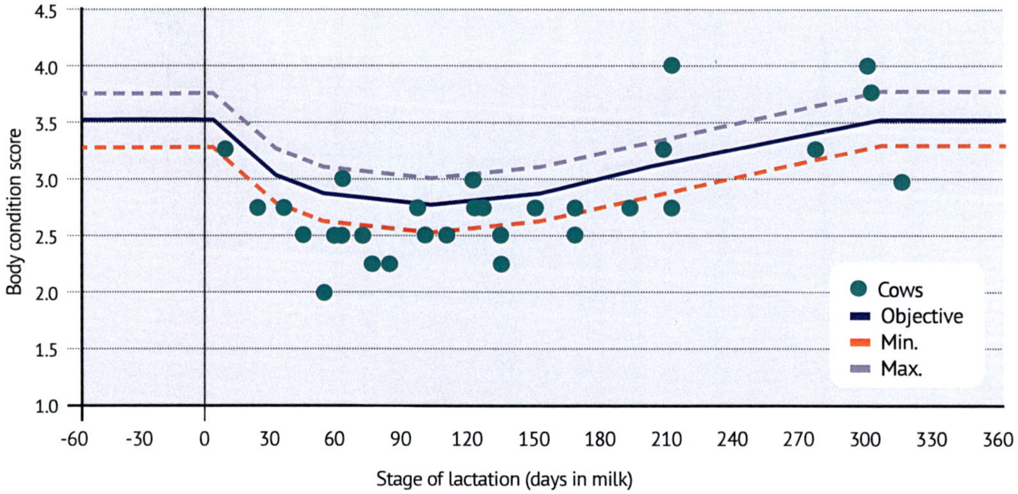

Case 2

This farm has 100 cows that are fed using the Unifeed system. Some animals are over 150 days in lactation and instead of recovering body reserves, are overly thin. These observations suggest poor feeding management during the postpartum period (Fig. 20).

Case 3

This is a farm with 50 cows fed using the Unifeed system and supplemented using the ACD system. Some of the cows are recently calved, but many of the animals are over 150 days in lactation and are overly thin, suggesting mismanagement or malfunction of the ACD system (Fig. 21).

Figure 20. Graphical representation of body condition scores in Case 2 as compared with recommended scores. Source: www.cowsulting.com.

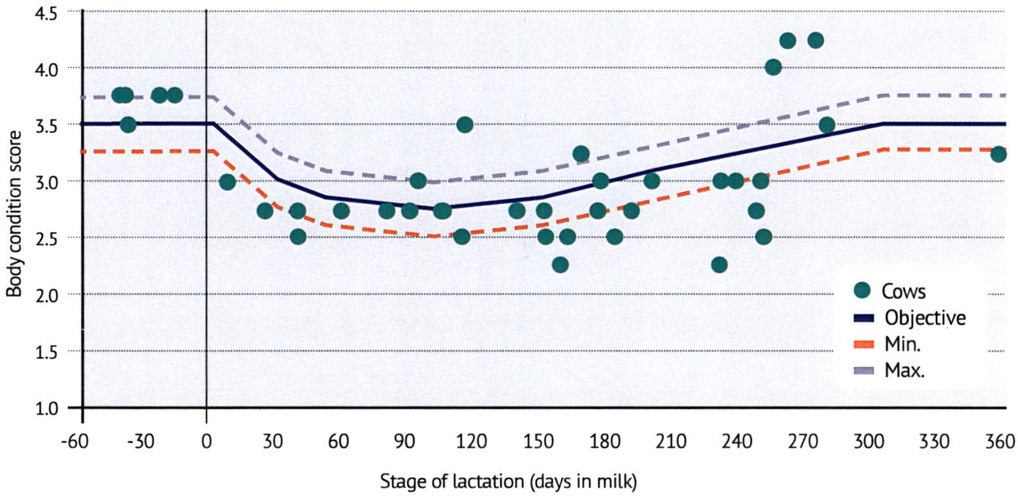

Figure 21. Graphical representation of body condition scores in Case 3 as compared with recommended values. Source: www.cowsulting.com.

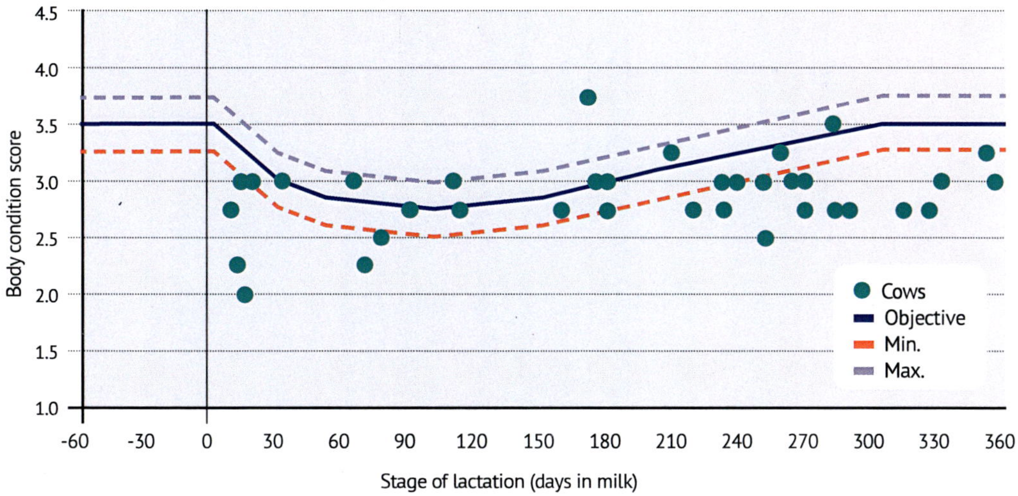

Case 4

This is a farm with 60 stall-fed cows that are fed on fodder and are supplemented with pelleted feed in the milking parlour. A large proportion of the cows on this farm are overly fat, and few thin cows are observed. This situation has affected the reproductive status of the herd (Fig. 22).

Figure 22. Graphical representation of body condition scores for Case 4 as compared with recommended values. Source: www.cowsulting.com.

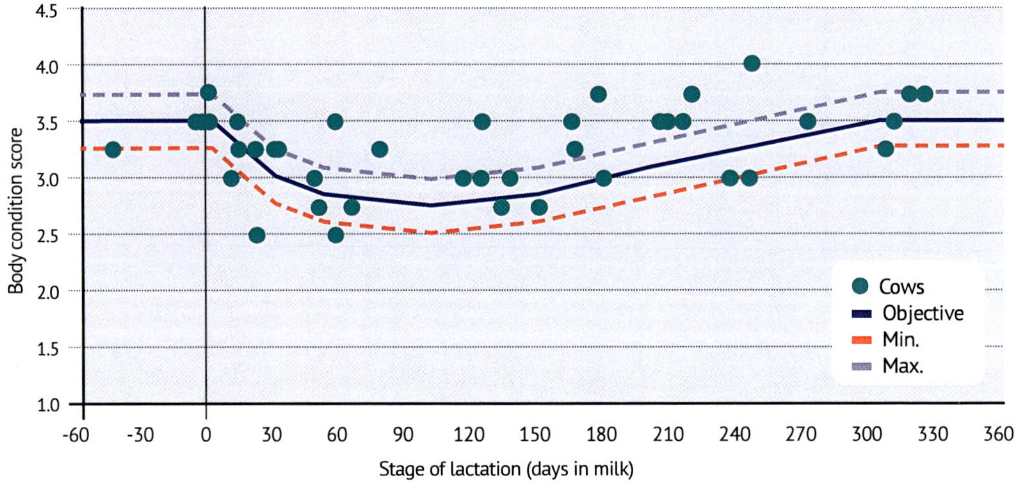

Case 5

This farm uses a Unifeed cart, which serves only poor quality grass silage. These cows lack sufficient energy in their ration, as evidenced by the high number of thin cows at any given stage of lactation (Fig. 23).

Figure 23. Graphical representation of body condition scores for Case 5 as compared with recommended values. Source: www.cowsulting.com.

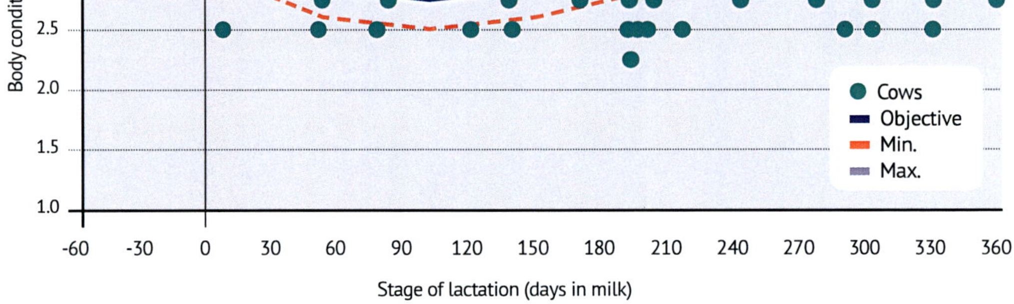

REMEMBER

The body condition of each cow should be assessed bearing in mind the following:

- The end of pregnancy is the best time to recuperate body condition.
- Ideally, the body condition score of a dry cow should neither increase nor decrease.

Changes in body condition

Even if a cow's BCS increases during the dry period, weight loss should not be induced as this can worsen the cow's metabolic problems. In these cases it is better to take preventative measures.

In cases in which BCS decreases during the dry period:

- Body condition can be somewhat restored by providing the cow with feed containing the appropriate amounts of fibre, energy, trace elements and vitamins.
- It is difficult to increase BCS by more than 0.5 points per month.
- If it appears that a cow will be overly thin at the time of calving, preventative measures such as those described above should be implemented. Furthermore, treatment should be individualised for each cow and their diet supplemented with a suitable feed.

Rations

If the average production of the farm, the milk quality (fat, protein and urea levels) and the lactation curve are considered when calculating the ration, it is likely that the resulting ration is appropriate. Accordingly, the ration designed by the computer programme will correspond with that which the farmer actually offers the cows, and the nutritional value of these rations will correspond with the predicted requirements of the cows. Nutritionists often check to ensure that the calculations are in agreement with the computer data, as this is more convenient than having to subsequently assess the ration requirements of each individual cow. Developing an adequate ration requires observation and interpretation of many signs displayed by the cows; the more attention given to the animals, the better the results. Establishing a good ration should thus be considered a starting point, after which cows must be closely monitored.

Case studies on ration management

Case 1

In the ration in this case, there are variations of almost 2.2 kg of dry matter/cow/day, from 13 to 18.5 kg of grass silage, and from 26 to 29 kg of corn silage, and cows consume 8.5-9 kg of mixed concentrates (Table 6). The ration consumed by the cattle on this farm corresponds with that which was initially calculated, and the number of rations provided is adequate. However, the person preparing the Unifeed cart is not sufficiently precise, and the quantities leaving the cart do not

Table 6. Example ration.

Date	Ration	Grass silage (GS)	GS/ cow	Corn silage (CS)	CS/ cow	Mix	Mix/ cow	Dry grass (DG)	DG/ cow	Leftover	Cart	Kg/ cow	Dry matter
01-11-07	60.00	1,030.00	17.17	1,745.00	29.08	550.00	9.17	45.00	0.75	0.00	3,370.00	56.17	22.71
02-11-07	65.00	1,200.00	18.46	1,700.00	26.15	570.00	8.77	50.00	0.77	A lot	3,520.00	54.15	21.98
03-11-07	60.00	1,100.00	18.33	1,750.00	29.17	565.00	9.42	35.00	0.58	100.00	3,450.00	57.50	23.21
04-11-07	60.00	800.00	13.33	1,700.00	28.33	520.00	8.67	30.00	0.50	0.00	3,050.00	50.83	20.57

fully correspond to those initially calculated, although the difference is generally fairly small.

The actual quantities of the rations consumed by the cows do not always correspond to those initially calculated by the nutritionist.

Behaviour of the cow towards its ration

It is important to evaluate cow behaviour after ration administration. Food should be made available to the animals for a period of 24 hours.

A protocol should be followed when evaluating the cow's response to its ration. Evaluation should begin one hour before the ration is administered. Scoring is conducted as follows:

- 0 = No feed is left in the trough. Increase ration by 5 %.
- 1 = Most of the trough is empty but some chunks of fodder remain. Increase ration by 2-3 %.
- 2 = Less than 2.5 cm of feed remains in the trough. Ration is correct.
- 3 = Between 5 and 7.5 cm of feed remains in the trough. Investigate possible causes.
- 4 = Over 50 % of feed remains in the trough. Investigate possible causes.
- 5 = Almost all of the feed remains in the trough. Investigate possible causes.

The way in which the cow sorts through the feed depends heavily on the treatment and chop length of the fodder, or more generally, the "mix quality". Laboratory analyses may help determine why food is being left in the trough by identifying the differences between the feed offered and that which is left untouched. Alternatively, the forage can be analysed using a particle separator 6 hours after administration and again the following day, and the results compared.

Another effective way to control fodder selection by cows is to analyse the type of cavities left in the forage as the cows feed.

- Well-defined cavities (Fig. 24) indicate that the cows do not need to be very selective.
- By contrast, if the animals are more selective, the forage will be well mixed, with fewer clear-cut cavities. The cow in Figure 25 is vigorously sorting through the forage, some of which has landed on its back.
- If the forage is not sufficiently chopped, cows select only the most desirable particles (Fig. 26). As a result, what the cow actually consumes differs considerably from the intended content of the ration.

Evaluation of cow manure

The degree of digestion of the total ration ingested by the cow is determined by both the degradability (passage through the rumen) and the digestibility (passage through the gut) of the nutrients. Thus, if any of the components of the ration are difficult to digest (e.g. corn silage that has been cut late), the total digestibility of the ration will be affected. Ration digestion can be determined by evaluating a cow's manure.

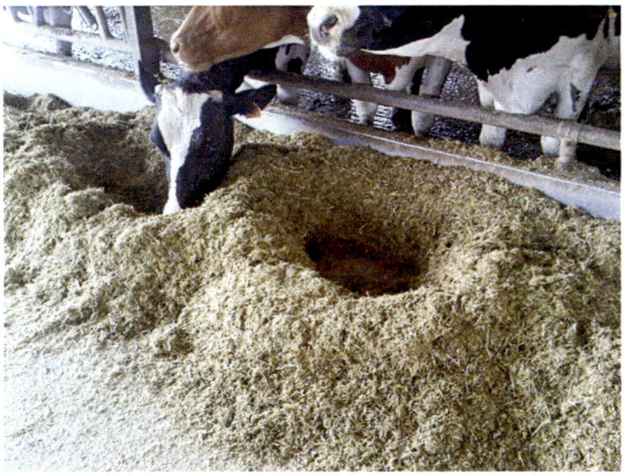

Figure 24. Marked cavities in the forage indicate that the cow does not need to sort much while feeding.

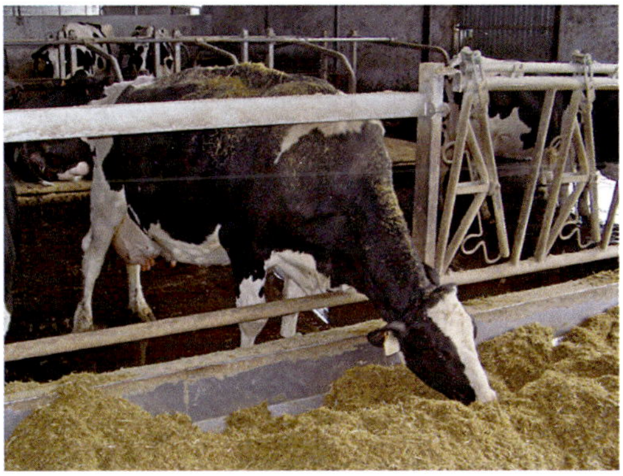

Figure 25. Cow sorting through fodder.

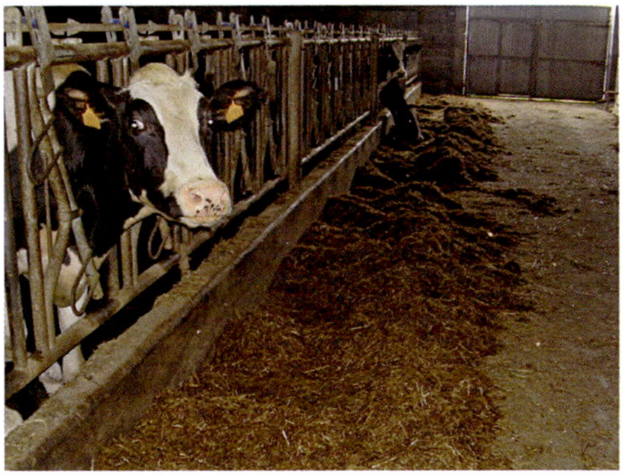

Figure 26. Fodder that has not been sufficiently chopped.

Case study on manure evaluation

Case 1

This farm has an ongoing acidosis problem due to the use of a ration consisting of freely available corn silage and concentrate containing excessive amounts of starch. Passing the faeces through a large-hole sieve (Fig. 27) reveals many residues of undigested corn. When an even finer sieve is used (Fig. 28), mucin strands can be seen, indicating damage to the walls of the large intestine. This may be due to an overly low pH of the digestive environment caused by excessive fermentation. If the intestine is damaged, the cow secretes mucin or fibrin to cover the damaged area of the intestinal mucosa.

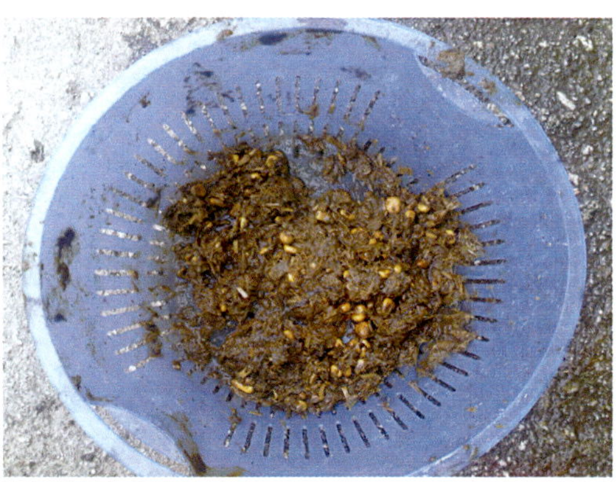

Figure 27. Manure evaluation using a large-pore sieve.

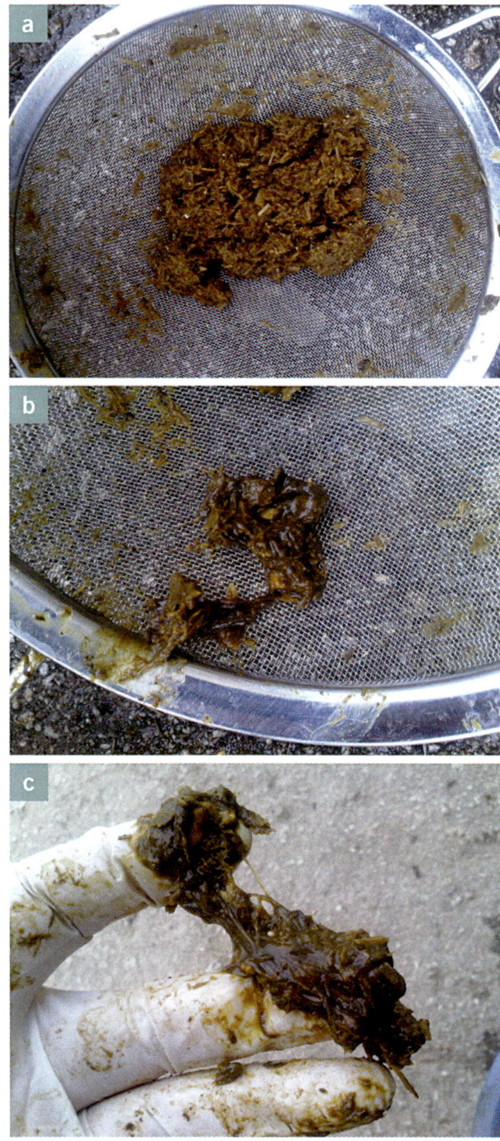

Figure 28. Manure evaluation using a fine sieve (b). Note the mucin strands (c).

5

Postpartum diseases

While each of the conditions described in this chapter could be more extensively discussed, our main goal is to emphasise the important interrelationships between the processes that occur around the time of calving. Each disorder is discussed briefly and concisely.

Hypocalcaemia, metritis and ketosis, all typical postpartum conditions, are the main diseases responsible for reproductive failure, culled cows during the peripartum period and poor reproductive rates on cattle farms. In near-chronological order, the main postpartum diseases encountered by veterinary surgeons specialising in dairy cattle are:

- Uterine prolapse.
- Hypocalcaemia.
- Retained placenta.
- Metritis.
- Ketosis.
- Left displaced abomasum (LDA).
- Mastitis.

Typically, both LDA and mastitis develop as a consequence of one or more of the diseases listed above.

Uterine prolapse

Externalisation or prolapse of the uterus is a serious disorder that can trigger a state of shock in the cow, as approximately 30 % of circulating blood is concentrated in the uterus at calving. Moreover, there is a high risk of uterine bleeding or tearing and of elongation of the uterus (the uterus weighs 20-35 kg at the time of calving), from which the cow may not recover.

The expulsion of urine is also impeded for the duration of the prolapse due to physical blockage of the urethra. Uterine prolapse usually occurs immediately after calving. The ambient temperature, location of calving and the time taken for the veterinary surgeon to intervene are key factors that influence the resolution of uterine prolapse (Fig. 1).

Aetiology

Uterine prolapse can occur due to:

- Dystocic calving: mainly posterior presentation of the calf, forced removal and uterine torsion.
- Concurrent diseases of the mother, e.g. hypocalcaemia.
- Calving on excessively inclined ground. This usually occurs when cows calve in mountainous areas.
- Excessive straining during expulsion of the placenta.

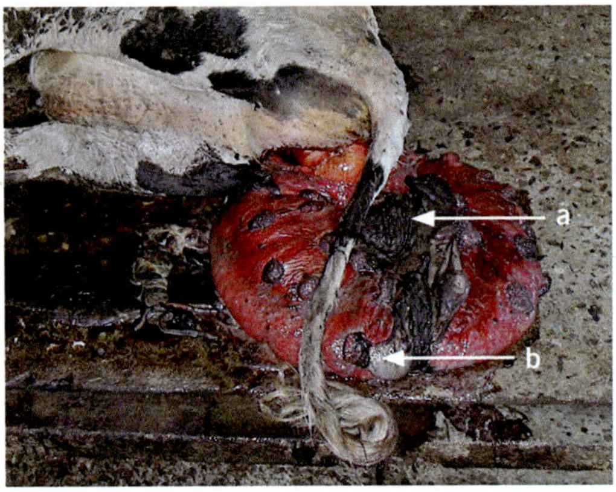

Figure 1. Cow with uterine prolapse. Note the faecal contamination (a) and the separation of the cotyledon from the caruncle (b). In this case, the placenta is almost detached.

Treatment

Before treating uterine prolapse, it is important to position and prepare the animal appropriately. It is essential that the necessary materials are prepared and that adequately qualified personnel are available to assist. Preplanning the treatment will ensure successful resolution in simple cases and will significantly decrease the likelihood of shock in more complicated cases. The aim is to minimise the number of manipulations required to reintroduce the uterus, as this organ is highly irrigated and in a fragile state after calving and due to the prolapse itself. We recommend the following protocol:

1. **Do not lift the cow if it is already lying down,** and ensure that it does not attempt to rise until the severity of the prolapse has been determined and the necessary material and personnel are prepared. Immobilise the cow in the position that best allows you to work.
2. **Make sure to have three or four competent assistants on hand.** The resolution of uterine prolapse in a cow can be a physically demanding job.
3. **Prepare the necessary material before the intervention.** It is essential to have warm water (40 °C) in a clean container, and some sheets or bath towels with which to cover the prolapsed uterus and prevent it from touching the ground, and one or two kilos of sugar.
4. **Perform a complete anamnesis of the case.** Make note of the calving number and any difficulties that have arisen during calving, the length of time since calving, and any action taken to date.
5. **Assess the general condition of the animal.** Check whether the cow has expelled the placenta, and determine whether there is an imminent risk of shock, hypocalcaemia or other complications. These data will complement the anamnesis.
6. **Administer the necessary drugs** before and after the intervention.
7. **Separate the placenta from the uterus.** First, wash the periphery of the vulva with iodine soap and tie the tail (which will be inert due to the epidural) forward. Before beginning the separation process, wash the uterus with iodine soap while visually inspecting and assessing its general appearance, colour, mucosal integrity and looking for any signs of injury. Each caruncle should be separated from its corresponding cotyledon with great care, starting with the gravid uterine sac and then moving on to the non-gravid uterine horn. The latter tends to be more difficult to handle as it is smaller and not usually exposed (i.e. it must be manipulated "blind"). Throughout the process, the uterus should be irrigated continuously with a solution of warm water in which sugar has been dissolved (1 kg sugar per 10 L water). This solution, together with drugs that prevent bleeding, helps to seal the exposed caruncles (Fig. 2).
8. **The uterus should be washed again after removal of the placenta.** Next, raise the cow on all fours, always supporting the uterus with

If the cow stands up, the assistants must lift the sheet or towel and support the weight of the uterus.

PHARMACOTHERAPY

- **Epidural anaesthesia:** lidocaine is administered as an epidural anaesthetic to attenuate contractions, which can significantly hamper reintroduction of the uterus. Administration of the epidural anaesthesia is delayed only if the animal needs to be lifted up first.
- **Uterine stimulants:** ergonovine or carbetocin are administered intravenously to induce uterine contractions and reduce the size of the organ, increasing its tone and preventing bleeding. The uterus is more manageable after treatment with these drugs, which also favour the expulsion of placenta if this has not already occurred.
- **Spasmolytic drugs in combination with xylazine:** this drug combination is administered once the uterus has been reintroduced.
- **Antibiotics:** the most commonly used antibiotics are penicillin + streptomycin and/or ceftiofur.
- **Other drugs:** the administration of calcium (hypocalcaemia), analgesics (pain) or saline (shock) may be necessary some cases. Continuous drug administration via a drip may also be required.

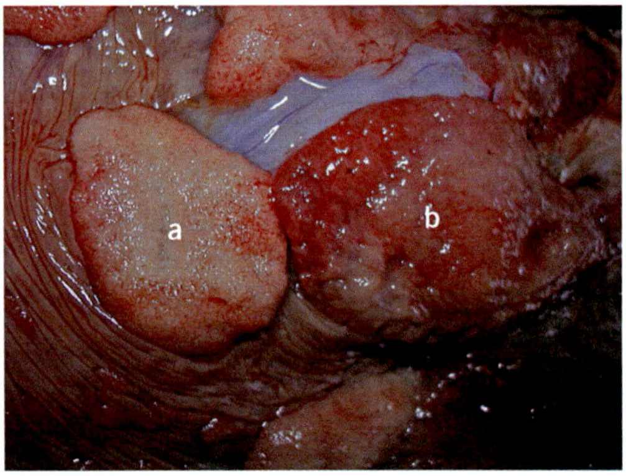

Figure 2. Recently cleaned, prolapsed uterus. The caruncle of the uterine horn (a) and the placental cotyledon (b) are in the process of separating.

a sheet or towel. Once the surrounding area is cleaned, the sheet or towel should be replaced with a fresh one moistened with water and iodine.

9. **Reintroduction of the uterus.** Start by applying light pressure to the uterus, towards the vulva, keeping the uterus slightly above the level of vulva throughout the procedure. The first portion to be reintroduced is the vagina. This manipulation is only effective if the cow is not experiencing intense contractions (although medicated, a certain degree of straining always occurs). To avoid damaging the uterus, it is essential to act with patience and the utmost care throughout the reintroduction process. Normally, it takes between five and 20 minutes to reintroduce 50 % of the uterus, after which the remaining portion enters with little resistance. Once the uterus is reintroduced, it is important to establish that the animal can urinate normally; if not, catheterisation will be required. If the cow is unable to stand up after reintroduction of the uterus, it should be placed in sternal recumbency with the hindlimbs apart and extended backwards so that the body weight is

supported by the knees (femorotibial joints). For ease of handling and to minimise stress, the cow should first be sedated (using a combination of xylazine and a spasmolytic) and using ropes, should be positioned to facilitate reintroduction of the uterus. After resolving the prolapse, the animal is placed in a sitting position and examined to ensure that the organ has been completely reintroduced. This can be done by introducing a sterilised glass bottle as deep as possible into the vagina.

10. Finally, it is recommended to suture **the vulva** with three or four U-stitches using polyamide 6 suture thread or vaginal tape and a Bühner needle (Fig. 3). It is important that the cow remains relaxed and calm after the intervention; a combined dose of xylazine and a spasmolytic should be administered and the cow placed it in a comfortable place where it can be easily monitored.

Cows that have experienced uterine prolapse should be examined within a few hours of treatment and should undergo further revision one month later to determine whether they can begin breeding again. It is important to closely monitor these animals to check that urination proceeds normally. If urination is impaired, the cow should be catheterised every eight hours.

Some cases of uterine prolapses are particularly complicated and can be fatal (e.g. cases involving vaginal and uterine rupture and concurrent intestinal prolapse). In these cases, the veterinary surgeon will often opt to euthanise the cow.

Hypocalcaemia

Hypocalcaemia is a metabolic disease associated with milk production and calving that is

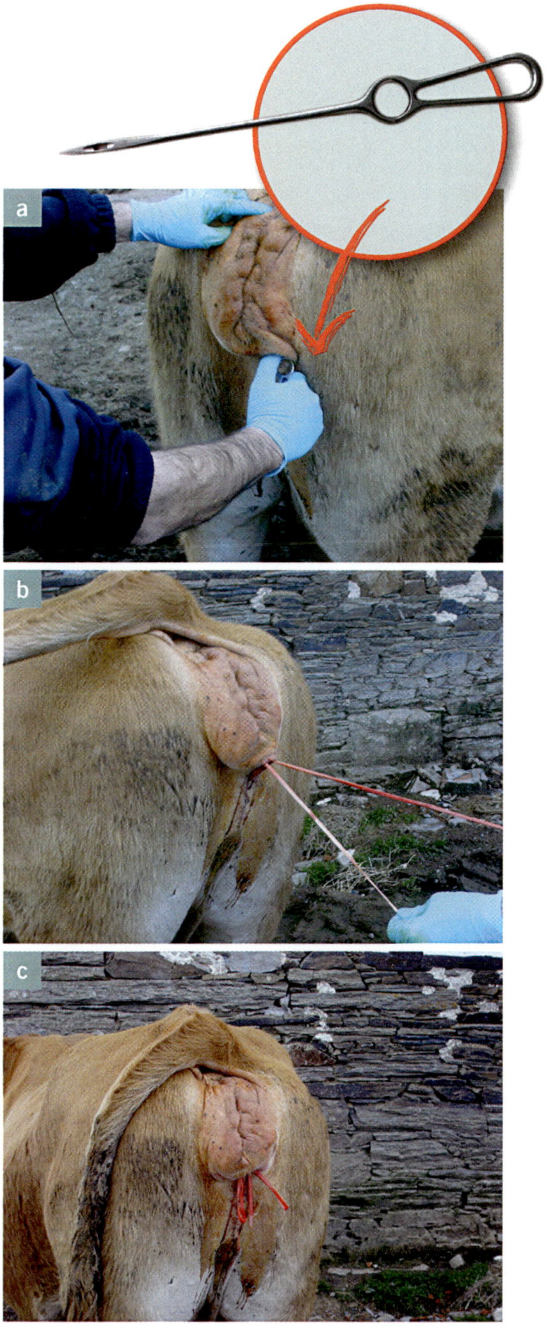

Figure 3. Suture of the vulva of a Rubia Gallega cow with uterine prolapse. The vet punctures the lips of the vulva with a Bühner needle, which has been threaded with vaginal tape (a). The vaginal tape is passed through both lips creating a circular closure (b). The ends of the tape are knotted to ensure closure of the vulva after prolapse (c).

characterised by low blood concentrations of calcium. While clinical hypocalcaemia is easily recognisable, the subclinical form is not, although both pose a high risk to the cow as they favour the development of other peripartum diseases and can affect reproduction.

Pathogenesis

Hypocalcaemia is caused by the abrupt changes experienced by the cow after calving. Colostrum contains twice as much calcium as normal milk, and milk in turn contains 10 times the concentration of calcium as blood. Accordingly, calcium requirements are increased substantially, even in the earliest stages of lactation.

Calcium metabolism is regulated by a homeostatic mechanism involving two hormones: PTH (parathyroid hormone) and calcitonin. PTH secretion is mediated by dietary calcium intake and the release of soluble calcium from the bones. The mobilisation of bone calcium is increased by slight acidification of the blood. Endogenous calcium levels depend on other factors such as the level of calcium in the diet, the digestibility of the ration, interactions with other minerals, vitamin D3 levels, age, calving number, twin pregnancy, and the feed supply system used.

During lactation, a cow loses 50-70 g of calcium per day.

It is very important that during the transition period the cow is provided with feed with a proper anion/cation balance, as an excess of cations favours the development of hypocalcaemia. The anion/cation balance is the most important factor influencing calcium metabolism, and must be considered in order to prevent disease.

Some degree of hypocalcaemia is normal in postpartum cows, and can even be considered physiological, but in other cases this disease manifests due to a failure to compensate for the significant changes in calcium metabolism that occur around calving.

Clinical signs

Hypocalcaemia usually occurs after calving, although it may occur earlier and affect the expulsion phase.

The clinical symptoms of hypocalcaemia can vary considerably, from mild cases associated with decreased body temperature, listlessness and reduced rumination, to more serious cases in which the cow remains prone, and repeatedly attempts to rise only for its posterior third to collapse. In even more extreme cases, the cow presents with hypothermia (< 37 °C), and lies on one side in a comatose state.

Subclinical hypocalcaemia, on the other hand, favours the development of other peripartum diseases and should also be prevented. The low concentration of calcium leads to a lack of muscle tone of the abomasum, uterus and teat sphincter, triggering conditions such as LDA, retained placenta, metritis and mastitis.

Treatment

Hypocalcaemia is treated by the intravenous administration of calcium, magnesium and

KEY POINTS

- In cows, the capacity to absorb calcium declines with age.
- Ideally, the prepartum period should have a low Ca^{2+}/P^{+} ratio.
- Calcium levels are significantly affected by diet. Keeping a cow grazing during the prepartum period may pose an additional risk, as this forage is rich in calcium.
- The presence of vitamin D3 in the diet promotes intestinal absorption of calcium from food.
- The ability to release soluble calcium from bone decreases with age, and is also dependent on PTH.
- PTH release is influenced by dietary levels of calcium: the less calcium in the diet, the more PTH is secreted.

phosphorus salts. Vitamin D, glucose and corticosteroids can also be administered. Treatment is administered for two or three days, depending on the severity of the disease. Administration can be intravenous (shock therapy), intramuscular, subcutaneous or oral. A satisfactory treatment response is obtained in a high percentage of cases of clinical hypocalcaemia. For a good outcome, it is essential to make a correct diagnosis early, to house the sick cow in an appropriate pen with a suitable bed during the recovery period and to ensure that the animal does not injure itself when attempting to stand while weakened by the disease. The recovery process is slower in cows that have a high percentage of body fat, as these animals have a greater risk of developing steatosis and other complications (see Case 6, p. 126).

Prevention

Prevention of hypocalcaemia:

- Reduce calcium intake during the prepartum period to stimulate PTH secretion.
- Control the anion/cation balance in the diet and neutralise excess cations in feed during the prepartum period by orally administering magnesium salts. This decreases metabolic alkalosis and triggers mild acidosis, which stimulates calcium mobilisation, although the use of these salts is limited by their unpalatability.
- Provide vitamin D3 to promote calcium absorption from food.
- Administer oral and injectable calcium a few hours before and immediately after calving.

Retained placenta

From the physiological point of view, placental retention indicates that calving has not been fully completed. The placenta is considered retained when 12 hours have passed since the time of delivery and the cow has not yet expelled the placenta and foetal membranes.

In cases of retained placenta, a certain amount of organic material stops receiving blood supply and "dies", and subsequently begins to decompose inside the uterus. A cow usually has between 80 and 120 placentomes (conjoined caruncles and cotyledons), which join the endometrium and the foetal membrane. These placentomes range in diameter from 10 cm in the gravid uterine horn to 2-4 cm in the non-gravid horn (Fig. 2).

Placental retention usually extends over several days (3-12 days). The placenta is normally expelled after nine or 10 days, either whole or in fragments, and is accompanied by a variable amount of fluid generated by concurrent metritis (Fig. 4). In fact, many cases of metritis are caused by complete or partial placental retention, with the dead tissue acting as an initial "broth" for the growth of microorganisms. If a cow exhibits clinical signs of metritis but placental retention cannot be confirmed, an ultrasound should be performed (Fig. 5).

Aetiology

Placental retention can be triggered by a variety of factors, including inadequate handling, which stresses cows (see Case 4, p. 114), mineral deficiencies, infectious diseases, twin calving, dystocia, and concurrent diseases. In any case, the impact of retained placenta on the farm should be assessed and compared with an acceptable mean rate (< 10 %).

After this initial evaluation, it is essential to identify the primary cause. For example, if a farm has a high percentage of twin calvings, the risk of retained placenta is higher. Similarly, decreases in the average gestation length on a farm imply an increased probability of placental retention. In the latter case, it is important determine the cause of the decrease in the average gestation length.

Clinical signs

The symptoms exhibited by a cow with retained placenta can vary considerably. In some mild cases, no fever is detected, and clinical signs, if present, usually resolve spontaneously in 9-10

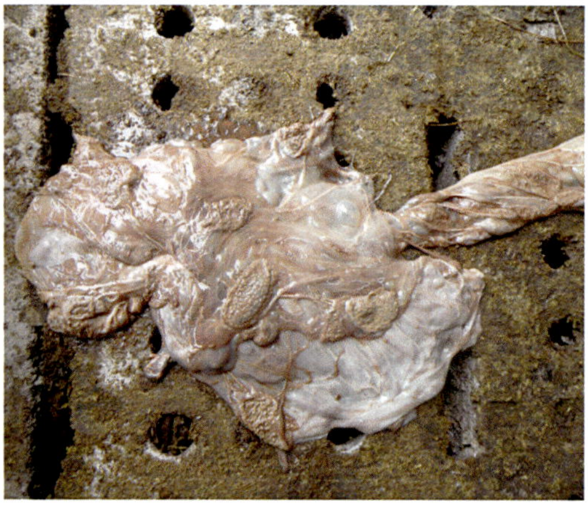

Figure 4. Unusual case in which the complete placenta was expelled nine days postpartum. The cotyledons are easily identifiable.

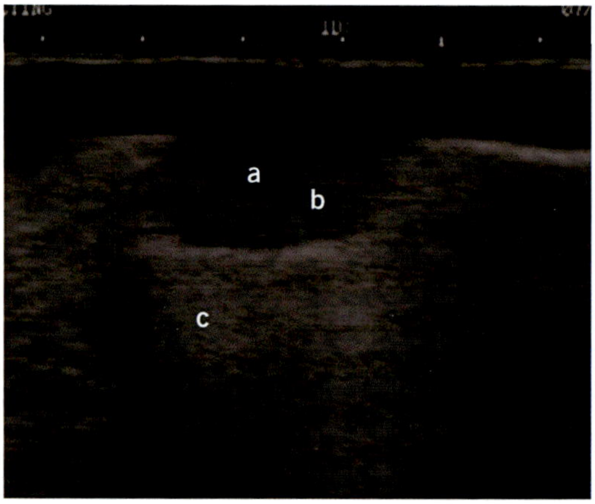

Figure 5. Ultrasound image of the uterus of a cow in which a caruncle (a), a cotyledon (b) and accumulated uterine fluid due to metritis (c) can be seen.

> Repeated cases of retained placenta on a farm may be an indication that something is wrong.

days, after the expulsion of the placenta and fluids, without requiring antibiotic therapy. In more severe cases, cows expel foul-smelling liquid and show clinical signs of toxaemia almost from the moment of calving until 12-15 days later. In many cases, the placenta per se is not expelled, but the cow expels tissue debris and purulent reddish brown exudate over the course of several days. Between these two extremes are a wide range of cases characterised by some degree of fever and deterioration in the cow's general health.

Some authors have suggested that placental retention leads to necrosis, uterine atony, oedema of the membranes, immature placentomes or placentitis. Placental retention frequently gives rise to metritis, which is discussed in the following section.

Treatment

The complex mechanism that mediates the separation of the caruncle from the cotyledon begins several hours before calving and involves neutrophils, enzymes, and contractile forces.

Retained placenta is usually treated with calcium, ergonovine and oxytocin. Although the expected result is not always achieved, it is worth persisting with these therapies designed to mobilise the retained membranes.

We do not recommend any manipulation of the placenta other than that required to confirm retention, as any attempt to remove the membranes can lead to the development of metritis. Any manipulation can facilitate the entry of germs and cause small lesions and tears in the lining of the uterus, making the organ more vulnerable and permeable to contaminants. In our experience, intrauterine treatments rarely resolve retained placenta and carry an added risk of contamination, although drainage of the uterus can be effective in cases of toxaemic metritis, as this treatment dilutes the contaminated contents of the uterus.

To treat retained placenta we recommend parenteral antibiotic therapy for 4-6 days, and monitoring of the overall status of the cow in case toxaemic metritis develops. If this occurs, NSAIDs and fluid therapy should also be administered. We usually administer natural prostaglandins on postpartum days 4, 8, 12 and 22, and follow-up after treatment. While other authors have argued against the effectiveness of prostaglandins so soon after calving, we have observed a favourable response to this treatment in terms of both uterine tone and fluid expulsion.

In summary, we recommend symptomatic treatment, which should be monitored daily, ensuring that the cow maintains a high dry matter intake, thereby preventing the onset of other conditions such as ketosis and LDA.

Prevention

Uterine atony should be treated preventatively, as this condition can trigger placental retention. Although only one of the possible causes of placental retention, uterine atony is the only condition that can be resolved in the short term.

The administration of selenium and vitamin E is also recommended on farms with a high rate of placental retention but no apparent infectious aetiology. In these cases, all factors relating to calving should be investigated to identify the cause of the high rate of placental retention.

> As there is no miracle treatment for this condition, retained placenta is best prevented by acting on the processes that occur around the time of calving.

Metritis

When cows recover after calving and undergo uterine involution, they are subjected to a contaminated environment, postpartum immunosuppression and stressful changes in housing and handling procedures. While the incidence of metritis varies between countries, geographic regions, and individual farms, studies of the prevalence of this disease in dairy cattle have generally revealed high levels of metritis and endometritis.

Metritis is defined as uterine inflammation resulting from infection with *E. coli, A. pyogenes* or *F. necrophorum*. This occurs during early lactation and affects all uterine layers. Effects include retained placenta, oedema, leukocyte infiltration and degeneration of the muscle layer of the uterus, which results in an increase in the size of the uterus and other general health problems.

Metritis can easily develop into **endometritis**, which has no clinical symptoms but has significant implications from a reproductive standpoint. In some cases, the inflammatory and infectious processes extend beyond the uterus, causing adhesions, abscesses, or inflammation of the surrounding tissue and viscera, which in turn can give rise to **perimetritis** or **parametritis**.

Aetiology

Various predisposing factors that favour metritis can have cumulative effects, increasing the chances of developing the disease:

- Retained placenta and associated risk factors.
- Dystocia (e.g. posterior presentation, corrective manipulations).
- Twin pregnancy.
- Miscarriage and/or stillbirth.
- Peripartum diseases that compromise the defences of the cow (e.g. hypocalcaemia, ketosis, LDA, lameness, mastitis).
- Age and calving number (higher values indicate a greater likelihood of developing metritis, although first-lactation heifers also tend to have a high incidence).
- Poor body condition (primarily high body condition score).

- Duration of dry period (longer dry periods increase the risk of metritis).
- Inadequate facilities.
- Improper bedding or inadequate hygiene in the calving area.
- Social stress or any kind of manipulation that can have immunosuppressive effects.

Clinical signs

The following is a quick and easy method for the classification of metritis. Using this method, the veterinary surgeon, farmer or qualified employee can group cows with metritis based on clinical features, act early and apply the most appropriate therapy in each case.

The clinical signs of the three types of **clinical metritis** shown in the diagram in Figure 6 are expressed in the first 21 days postpartum. All three forms are characterised by an increase in the size of the uterus and the expulsion of foul-smelling liquid through the vagina. The main differences between the different types of metritis are:

- **Grade 1:** no systemic signs of illness.
- **Grade 2 (puerperal metritis):** the cow expels foul-smelling discharge from the vagina beginning around postpartum days 3-5, has a temperature between 39.5 °C and 40.5 °C and presents systemic signs of illness to varying degrees.
- **Grade 3 (toxaemic metritis):** the cow expels foul-smelling discharge from the vagina, presents severe systemic signs of illness and has a high risk of mortality. The body temperature of the cow may be normal or even reduced due to toxaemia. Symptoms include depression, frequent lying down, and tachycardia.

Figure 6. Diagram showing the three types of clinical metritis.

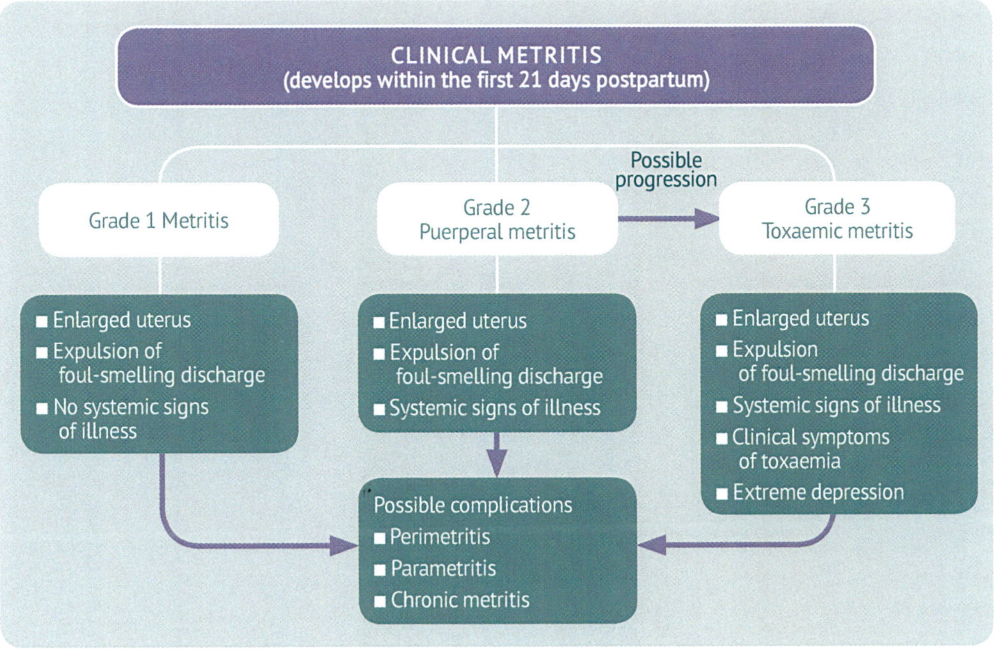

Toxaemic metritis may develop from puerperal metritis that is complicated or not properly treated, but in some cases is directly triggered by a combination of negative factors before or during calving, and may even appear the day after calving (Fig. 7).

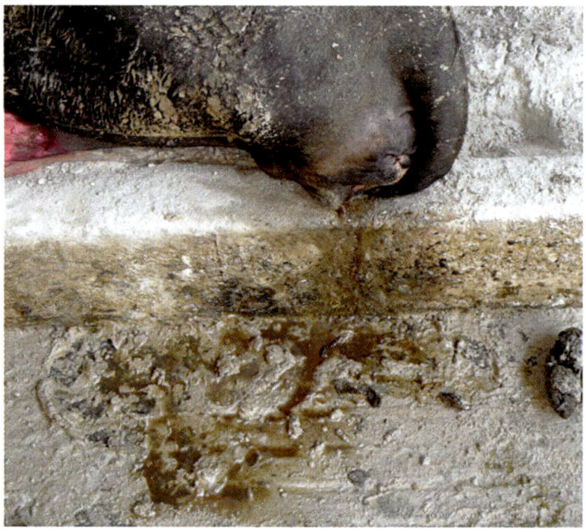

Figure 7. Cow expelling dark brown, foul-smelling discharge characteristic of toxaemic metritis.

Endometritis develops after postpartum day 21 and is the logical progression of prior metritis, regardless of the initial degree of metritis. This condition has significant reproductive effects, although it tends not to affect productivity. It is important to remember that this condition originates from undiagnosed, untreated or uncured metritis.

Endometritis can be classified as:

- Clinical: the cow produces odourless discharge and exhibits little thickening of the uterus.
- Subclinical: the cow produces no discharge, and diagnosis is thus more difficult.

Pyometra is another type of disease that can develop from prior metritis and is characterised by the accumulation of purulent material in the uterus and the presence of a corpus luteum in the ovary (Fig. 8). Cows with pyometra rarely present clinical symptoms, except for vaginal discharge and in some cases a closed cervix.

Figure 8. Diagram describing endometritis and pyometra.

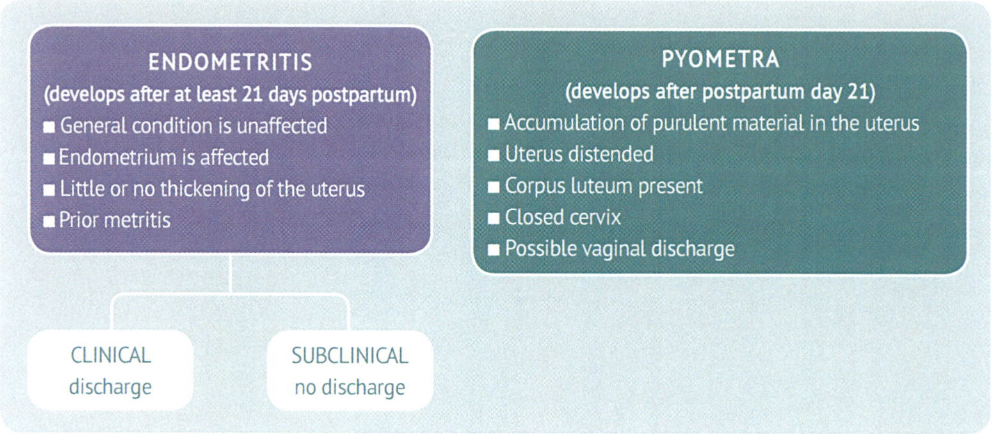

Diagnosis

The diagnosis of metritis is based on the detection of clinical signs. Particular attention should be paid to early diagnosis of metritis types 2 and 3 to prevent future complications due to concurrent diseases. Sick animals should be monitored to prevent possible endometritis. Implementing a protocol to monitor recently calved cows will significantly facilitate early diagnosis of these processes. Cases of recurring subclinical endometritis can be easily diagnosed by ultrasound.

Cows with severe metritis require daily monitoring to evaluate disease progression and treatment efficacy.

Treatment

The objective of **prostaglandin** administration is to promote the complete expulsion of the inflammatory or infectious material (uterine fluids) in cows with metritis. In our experience, these drugs promote the discharge of uterine fluids and a significant increase in uterine tone in most cases. We administer prostaglandins on postpartum days 4, 8, 12 and 22, although additional doses may be subsequently administered if necessary.

Ergonovine, **oxytocin** or **carbetocin** are used in cases in which the cervix remains open 24 hours after calving, permitting vaginal examination. This scenario occurs in cows that are predisposed to puerperal or toxaemic metritis, and thus special care is advised when performing the anamnesis, especially in cases in which several risk factors converge (e.g. hypocalcaemia, twin pregnancy, high calving number).

Parenteral antibiotic therapy is essential in cases of clinical metritis grades 2 and 3. In these cases, a combination of penicillin and streptomycin is typically administered, although other antibiotics may be also administered depending on the presence of concurrent diseases.

NSAID administration is also important to control the temperature increase in cows with grade 2 or 3 clinical metritis.

Complementary **supportive therapy** should cover the treatment requirements of any concurrent diseases (e.g. calcium, glucose, choleretics, methionine, vitamins, compounds that increase triglyceride mobilisation) as well as toxaemia (e.g. hypertonic fluid therapy, oral hydration, supplements to promote the growth of ruminal flora).

We do not recommend manually removing the foetal membranes or performing uterine lavage for curative purposes. However, we recommend a uterine lavage to remove or dilute the accumulated liquid in the uterus, after epidural anaesthesia: we introduce about 2-3 litres of warm saline into the uterus and then remove as much of the liquid as possible. In our experience, it is best to perform this technique between 3 and 6 days after diagnosis of toxaemic metritis and the initiation of drug therapy (Fig. 9). Early diagnosis and treatment of metritis can significantly increase profitability, as it avoids or reduces the risk of future complications due to other diseases associated with the peripartum period.

Prevention

To prevent the occurrence of metritis, or to determine whether a cow requires preventative or curative treatment, it is important to regularly monitor the following parameters:

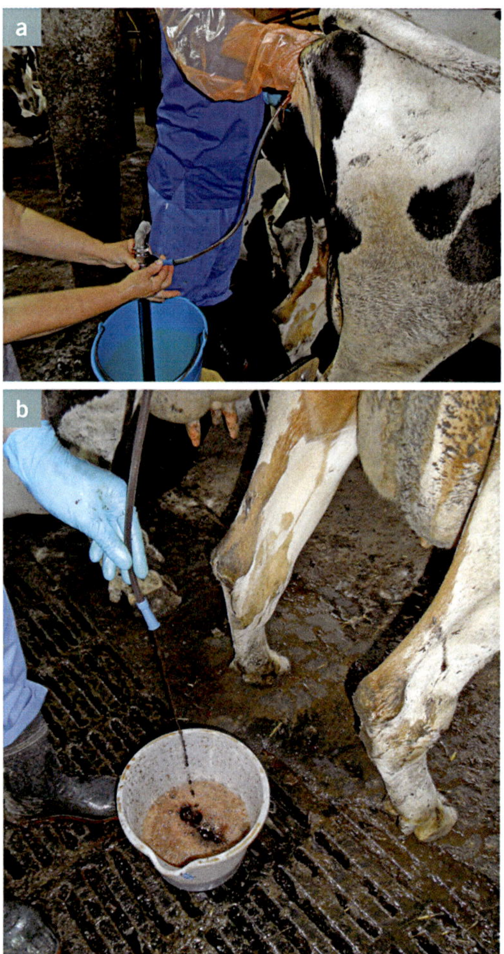

Figure 9. Uterine lavage as part of the treatment of a cow with metritis. The purpose is to dilute the contents of the uterus and favour the elimination of the greatest possible amount of fluid.

- **The degree of immunity of the cows**
  Feeding and handling during the antepartum and postpartum periods greatly influence the degree of immunity of a cow.
  - The diet during the transition period should contain appropriate amounts of calcium (to prevent hypocalcaemia), selenium and vitamins A and E. Moreover, the ration should be palatable and balanced in nutrients and should contain a high proportion of dry matter.
  - It is important to establish preventative measures to avoid ketosis; this disease has significant immunosuppressive effects in cows.
  - Feeding and drinking troughs and resting areas (bedding) must be correctly sized and easily accessible.
- **Hygiene and comfort in the calving area**
  Particular attention should be paid to the hygiene of the bedding, ventilation and the density of cows to avoid stressing pregnant cows. The calving area should be quiet and easily accessible to allow unintrusive monitoring of the mother.
- **The personnel assisting calving**
  The personnel assisting calving should be aware that good hygiene during calving is

> The ideal situation is that the cow reaches the moment of calving with a BCS between 3 and 3.5 and does not experience any abrupt changes in BCS during the dry period.

ACCORDING TO STUDIES BY OTHER AUTHORS:

- 1/3 of cows diagnosed with metritis remain empty at 300 days in milk.
- 50 % of cows suffer subclinical endometritis between 35 and 60 days in milk.

essential and should know to intervene only when necessary.

Other recommendations: use sanitised material, disposable gloves and wash the perineal area with soapy water and iodine before any intervention.

- **Postpartum monitoring**

Important postpartum data should be logged on a record sheet; these data are useful to conduct objective monitoring and establish protocols. The approach taken will be influenced by factors such as the number of animals per farm, the ability to create batches of animals, and the availability and experience of personnel.

A monitoring protocol should be established for the first 15 days after calving, except in cases of disease that necessitate longer surveillance. The following parameters should be monitored and recorded:

- Temperature.
- Rumen fill.
- Behaviour (activity, appetite, rumination, etc.).
- Progression of daily production.
- Vaginal secretions and discharges.
- Body condition.
- Ketone bodies (in urine) and beta-hydroxybutyrate (BHB, in blood or milk).
- pH.

All data gathered should be filed electronically to assess the progression of the herd and compare with other groups or farms.

Another type of record sheet can be used to record the most relevant data for each cow. Each page should identify the animal and include its medical history, daily production data (number of milkings, milking volume), health status (temperature, ketone bodies, BHB, urinary pH, behaviour, rumen fill) and information on any therapies or treatments that have been applied (start and end dates) (Table 1).

Ketosis

Ketosis, both clinical and subclinical, can have a significant impact on cow fertility, delaying ovulation and thus also affecting the likelihood of becoming pregnant.

Aetiology

From the beginning of the lactation period until peak production, the cow undergoes an inevitable "physiological" loss of body condition accompanied by increases in beta-hydroxybutyrate (BHB) levels. This occurs because the female must mobilise her fat reserves to provide the necessary energy to produce milk, resulting in an overall negative energy balance (NEB). At the same time, the female experiences a certain degree of hypoglycaemia (insulin levels are especially low at the beginning of lactation). Clinical ketosis will occur if this situation persists over time or if other conditions

Table 1. Model data sheet for monitoring cows after calving.

MONITORING OF RECENTLY CALVED COWS (SERVEPO SLP)							
Ear tag =	L (Lactation No./calving number) =				BCS (Body condition score) =		
Eutocic delivery? =		RP (retained placenta) =					
Day of delivery =	Number of days exceeding 9 months of gestation = ± 275 days						
Dry days =	Calving interval =				Dry period OK? =		
Farm =							
Day	**Examination and treatment**	**Milking**	**Temp.**	**Milk**	**Total**	**Other values**	
DAY 1		AM				BHB	
						BCS	
		PM				pH	
DAY 2		AM				BHB	
						BCS	
		PM				pH	
DAY 3		AM				BHB	
						BCS	
		PM				pH	
DAY 4		AM				K	
						BCS	
		PM				pH	
DAY 5		AM				BHB	
						BCS	
		PM				pH	
DAY 6		AM				K	
						BCS	
		PM				pH	
DAY 7		AM				BHB	
						BCS	
		PM				pH	
DAY 8		AM				BHB	
						BCS	
		PM				pH	
DAY 9		AM				BHB	
						BCS	
		PM				pH	
Treatment withdrawal date							

prevent a rapid increase in dry matter intake (DMI), which provides the energy and nutrients required for the production and maintenance of recently calved animals.

Pathogenesis

The pathogenesis of ketosis has a biochemical basis (Fig. 10). In the liver, the metabolism of fat (triglycerides) occurs via three possible pathways.

1. Accumulation of non-esterified fatty acids (NEFA) due to the mobilisation of the fat reserves of the animal, which triggers hepatic steatosis.
2. Triglycerides are oxidised and form an intermediate compound (acetyl coenzyme A), which in turn can be oxidised very efficiently in the presence of oxaloacetate to release energy and CO_2, or less efficiently in the absence of oxaloacetate to release BHB (the main ketone body).
3. If liver triglycerides are esterified, they are transformed and leave the liver as very low density lipoproteins (VLDLs).

Pathways 2 and 3 are physiological and do not induce disease, but are limited by the availability of the necessary precursors. Inactivation of pathways 2 and 3 results in the activation of pathway 1, increasing the risk of ketosis.

Possible means of preventing ketosis include:

- Mobilising less body fat.
- Maximising the efficiency of the pathways that "burn" fats and the availability of essential precursors.

In short, the liver acts as a "funnel" for triglycerides generated by the mobilisation of the cow's fat reserves. The physiological pathways that mediate the metabolism of fatty acids (triglycerides) involve oxidation and esterification, generating CO_2 and energy or very low density lipoproteins, respectively. However, these routes are limited by the availability of the necessary precursors. Thus, when these precursors are exhausted, pathological pathways are activated, which generate toxic products

Figure 10. Diagram showing the metabolic pathways of fatty acids in the liver at the time of calving.

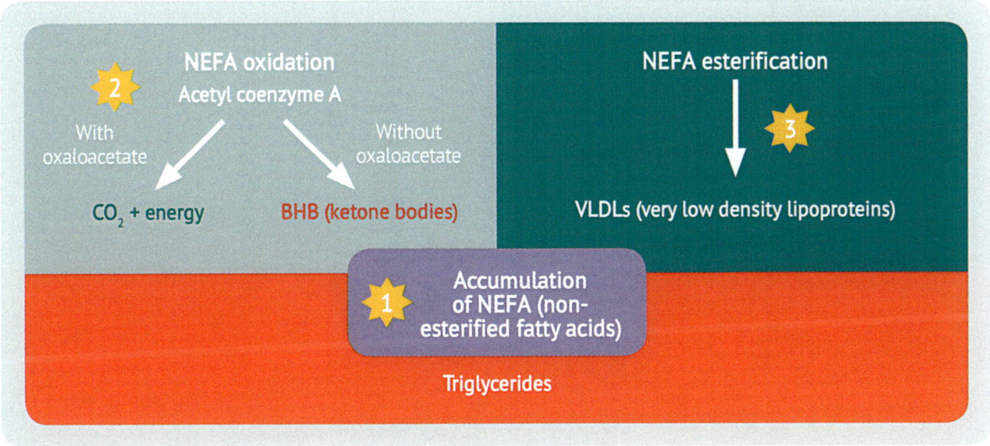

(ketones) or induce the accumulation of triglycerides in the liver, further promoting the mobilisation of fat reserves (Fig. 11).

Clinical signs

The main signs of primary **clinical ketosis** are loss of appetite and decreased production. If the ketosis is secondary, other symptoms of the primary disease (e.g. lameness, LDA, metritis) may also be observed. Nervous ketosis is quite rare and is easily identifiable. Subclinical ketosis is closely associated with NEB. In the early stages of lactation, nutrient intake is insufficient to meet the high energy demands required for milk production. The time taken to reach peak production will determine the future lactation curve and the total production of the cow.

This **subclinical disease** favours the development of other diseases (LDA, mastitis, increased number of days open) and can even be fatal, and thus has a significant economic impact on the farm, in addition to delaying the next reproductive cycle of affected females.

Diagnosis

Ketosis is diagnosed by the detection of characteristic clinical signs (loss of appetite and decreased production) and the presence of ketones in the urine, milk or blood.

It is important to be aware of the percentage of cases of subclinical ketosis on a farm and to monitor NEB in individual cows:

- Results of the analysis of prepartum **NEFA levels**. These can predict the degree of ketosis and NEB, both in individuals and in the herd as a whole.

Ideally:
NEFAs should be < 0.3 mEq/L during the last 14 days before calving.

Figure 11. Diagram showing the "funnel" effect of the liver when metabolising triglycerides produced by the mobilisation of the fat reserves of the cow.

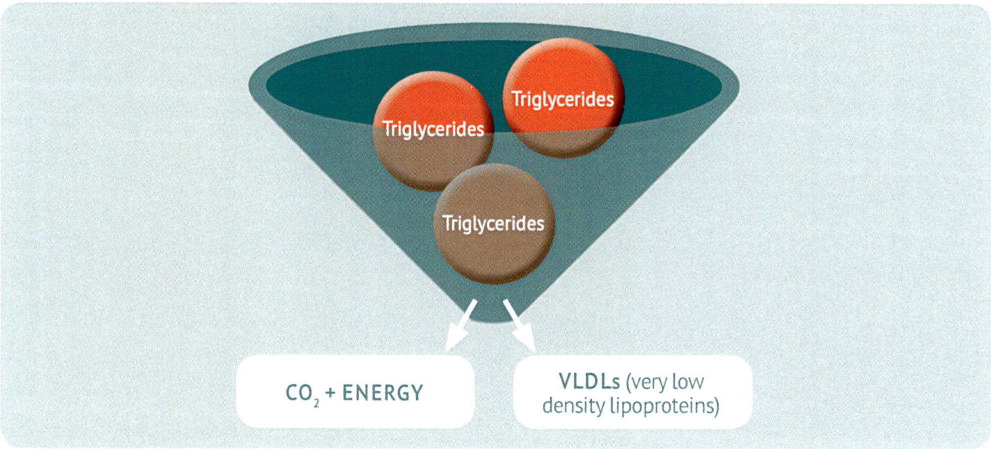

Clinical signs of ketosis appear when the BHB concentration exceeds 1.4 mmol/L.

- Results of the postpartum **NEFA and/or BHB** analyses serve as predictors of the degree of ketosis and NEB.

Ideally:
NEFAs < 0.7 mEq/L in the first 14 days after calving
BHB < 1.2-1.4 mmol/L in the first 14 days after calving

These tests should always be performed taking into account the clinical signs at the exact moment of testing, and the quantity and degree of preservation of the sample analysed. The results obtained after analysing the herd will indicate whether changes in diet and/or handling are necessary.

If higher than recommended values are obtained before calving, the veterinary surgeon should review the protocols used for drying-off, calving and postpartum care. If higher than recommended values are obtained only in the postpartum period, the vet should focus on the management of calving and postpartum care.

Treatment

Ketosis is treated by intravenous glucose administration in order to correct anorexia as soon as possible and to provide the precursors necessary to reactivate the physiological fat metabolism pathways. Therapy should be maintained until the cow fully recovers its appetite and ketonuria and/or BHB levels in urine normalise for at least three days after the last intravenous treatment. Finally, it should be established that the animal has regained both its appetite and level of production. Upon ending intravenous treatment, we recommend oral administration of glucose precursors (propylene glycol).

Intravenous glucose administration can vary in quantity, concentration and frequency. It is usually administered every 12 or 24 hours, and can be combined with amino acids, calcium, corticosteroids, and vitamins, or with choleretic or cholagogue substances (e.g. menbutone, phenoxymethyl propionic acid).

In cases of secondary ketosis, it is essential to assess the prognosis of the primary disease and to treat it if necessary.

Prevention

The main targets to prevent ketosis are the pathways that mediate the metabolism of non-esterified free fatty acids in the liver (Fig. 10):

1. **Moderate the arrival of NEFAs to the liver**
   - Ensure that animals are comfortable in order to maintain high intake (intake may be reduced at this time). Ensure that the cows are consuming their daily ration of quality feeds.
   - Provide cows with a ration containing an energy density that corresponds to the production level of the farm.

INTRAVENOUS ADMINISTRATION

The mammary vein of first-lactation heifers is less visible than that of older cows, as this vessel has not yet borne the burden of multiple lactations. This may hinder infusion via the **mammary vein**, leading to certain problems if repeated applications are required or if large volumes of fluid need to be administered.

The surrounding area should be disinfected before puncturing the vein. This also will make the blood vessel more visible. Always insert the needle in the direction of the blood flow so that drugs enter the bloodstream more easily and to avoid possible fluid backflow or extravasation (Fig. 12).

Extravasation of fluid containing 40-50 % glucose is highly irritating, and is likely to cause phlebitis, which in many cases becomes the primary disease (Fig. 13).

The jugular vein is an alternative route of intravenous drug administration, as long as the animal is adequately restrained and the needle is introduced in the direction of venous blood flow.

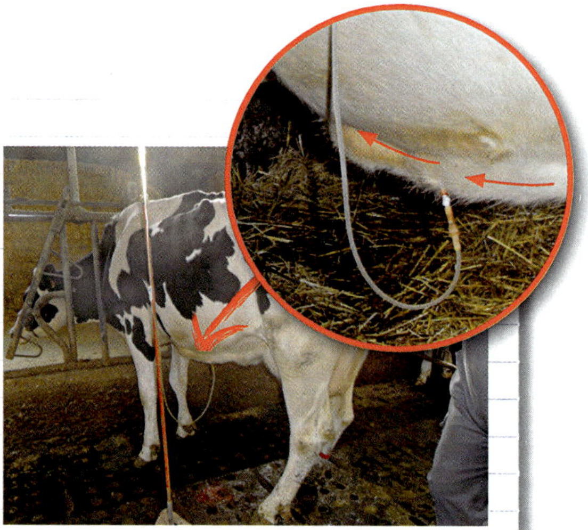

Figure 12. When performing venipuncture, the needle should be introduced in the direction of the blood flow to prevent reflux of the administered drug.

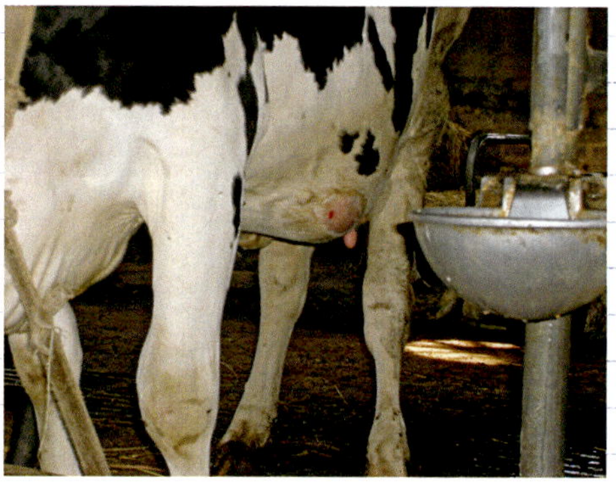

Figure 13. Phlebitis in a cow mammary vein due to extravasation of a 50 % glucose solution.

- Supplement the ration with calcium propionate, propylene glycol or glycerol.
- Prevent lipomobilisation by administering nicotinamide or nicotinic acid.

2. Enhance NEFA oxidation in the liver

- Enrich the cows' feed with the amino acids methionine and lysine. These act as substrates for the synthesis of carnitine, which plays an important role in fatty acid oxidation and favours NEFA metabolism.
- Orally administer oxaloacetate precursors (e.g. calcium propionate). The presence of oxaloacetate allows efficient oxidation of NEFAs, generating CO_2 and energy, whereas its absence results in ineffective oxidation and the production of toxic products (e.g. ketone bodies).

3. **Promote the elimination of fats such as VLDLs.**
   - The esterification of fatty acids is dependent on the enzyme phosphatidylcholine. Synthesis of this enzyme requires amino acids such as methionine and choline. The ration provided to the cows can be enriched with methionine and choline chloride to promote the direct production of phosphatidylcholine. Both these substances should be administered with a protective coating to prevent their degradation in the rumen.

> Although LDA can occur at any stage of lactation, it is more common in the early postpartum period.

Left displaced abomasum

Left displaced abomasum (LDA) is the most important secondary disease in the postpartum cow. Any alteration or disease that can impair the cow's appetite can lead to LDA within just a few hours.

Pathogenesis

Expulsion of the calf leaves a large space within the abdomen. Accordingly, the risk of LDA increases in the days after calving. Dry matter intake is also reduced at this time, and the potential consequences of concurrent diseases must also be considered. These include smooth muscle atony due to hypocalcaemia; apathy; decreased ingestion caused by concurrent processes (mainly metritis and ketosis); and other factors that cause stress and can decrease appetite, such as mastitis, lameness, and twin calving (Fig. 14).

LDA can also affect dry cows; in these cases LDA is usually caused by feeding errors, or changes in the locomotor system, especially if the disease in question, in addition to causing loss of appetite, forces the cow to spend long periods lying on its right flank.

The abomasum is located ventrally within the abdomen, and any of the causes listed above can trigger its displacement leftward. The presence of gas in the abomasum further exacerbates this displacement, causing the abomasum to rise along the left abdominal wall and to

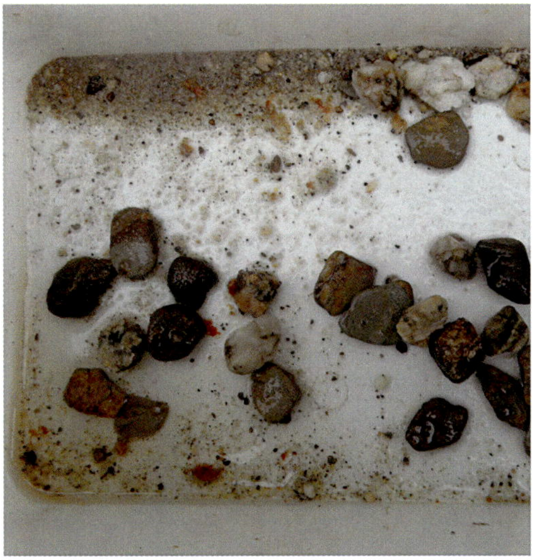

Figure 14. Many diseases of the peripartum period can result in LDA, although other causes can also trigger this disorder. In this case, the cow swallowed stones while feeding, resulting in obstruction of the pylorus and subsequent LDA.

sit medial to the rumen and lateral to the spleen and costal arch. In cases in which the cow stops eating, the size of the abomasum may exceed that of the rumen due to the accumulation of gases.

Clinical signs

The clinical signs of LDA are similar to those of the other conditions previously described, which often trigger this disease. These clinical signs include apathy, a sudden decrease in production, and secondary ketosis (which may be the trigger), in addition to other symptoms specific to the primary diseases that have triggered LDA.

In some cases, the cow will alternate between craving for food and periods of no appetite. Levels of accumulated gas decrease during these periods of craving, allowing relatively normal digestive functioning. However, constant ketosis caused by these continuous changes in appetite prolongs the situation and can in turn promote the development of other diseases.

Diagnosis

LDA can be easily diagnosed by auscultation combined with percussion and succussion of the abdomen in the area of the abomasum. An exploratory laparotomy is not usually required to reach a definitive diagnosis.

In some cases of LDA, the abomasum adopts a ventral position, while in others it is located dorsally and is highly compressed. Laparotomy is rarely necessary to confirm or rule out this condition.

Treatment

Given that surgical intervention is required in 95 % of cases of LDA, we recommend planning surgery from the outset. In cases involving another predominant disease, such as ketosis or hypocalcaemia, conservative treatment should first be initiated to deal with the primary disease and to provide a margin of about 24 hours before surgery.

Cases in which LDA is caused by another evident condition can sometimes be resolved by rolling the cow to correct the position of the abomasum. The use of this conservative treatment in appropriate cases has a success rate of 10-15 % (without recurrences).

Rolling procedure

Before starting the rolling procedure the animal should be tranquilised and cast on its right flank. Next, tie the forelimbs and hindlimbs and place the cow in a supine position. Once in this position, gently sway the cow from left to right while massaging the ventral abdomen.

This should move the abomasum from the left side of the abdomen to the upper middle area and finally to the right side. In some cases, a tractor or a shovel can be used to move or change the position of the cow once it has been lain down. After establishing that the abomasum is correctly positioned (on the right side of the abdomen) by auscultation, the animal should be cast on its left flank. The legs are then untied and the position of the viscera is verified again by auscultation/percussion once the animal is on all fours.

Before beginning the rolling procedure, it is essential to begin treatment of the primary disease that triggered LDA. If the abomasum remains in the correct physiological position 24 hours after rolling, the animal should be monitored and treatment of the primary disease continued. If LDA recurs, surgical treatment should be attempted, unless it is decided to euthanise the animal.

Surgery

LDA can be resolved surgically using three different approaches:

- Paramedian approach.
- Right flank approach.
- Left flank approach.

Paramedian approach

This approach requires general and local anaesthesia. The cow is cast on its right flank, and the forelimbs and hindlimbs bound. It is then placed in a near-supine position, ensuring that the abdomen remains conveniently accessible for surgery. Normally, by placing the cow in a supine position, the abomasum returns to its correct physiological position (rolling procedure). The head of the cow should remain to the left of the veterinary surgeon.

An incision is made in the right flank, about 15 cm behind the xiphoid process and parallel to and 5-10 cm from the linea alba. After opening the abdomen, the abomasum is punctured to remove accumulated gases, if necessary, which makes for easier handling. Next, the veterinary surgeon locates the greater curvature, the omentum and the wall of the abomasum, and massages the omasum.

From this point on, surgical techniques tend to vary: the omentum may be attached to the peritoneum and the muscular wall; the omentum may be alternated with the peritoneum, introducing non-perforating sutures in the abomasum; continuous sutures or individual stitches may be used. Finally, the muscle layer and the skin are closed over. After surgery, the cow should be housed in a clean and secluded place. The progression of the wound and the recovery of the animal should be closely monitored.

The paramedian approach is a safe method because it fixes the abomasum in its natural position and subsequent recurrence is rare. The disadvantages of this surgical technique are that it is long and laborious, and requires several assistants and a suitable place in which to cast the cow.

Right flank approach

This approach requires local anaesthesia; either an inverted "L" block or a proximal or distal paravertebral block. The method of administering the anaesthetic depends on the preference of the vet for one method or the other, and specific features of the cow that may affect administration (e.g. excessive body fat). An incision is made in the right flank, about 10 cm caudal to the last rib. Upon accessing the abdomen, the diagnosis is confirmed and the absence of adhesions verified. The peritoneal fluid should also be examined to look for the possible presence of fibrin, which can indicate other abdominal processes or damage to the integrity of the abomasum. Different approaches can be used to reposition the abomasum.

We recommend sliding the hand across the abdominal floor, past the linea alba and up along the left wall to locate the left flank. Contact with the parietal peritoneum should be maintained at all times. If the rumen obstructs the surgeon during this procedure, it can be pulled back towards the surgeon. Upon palpating the abdominal wall of the left flank, the surgeon raises their forearm, positioning it above the abomasum, and pushes down gently with the hand and forearm. When the abomasum is in a ventral position, it is then moved across the linea alba towards the right side. The last step is to massage the abomasum upward towards the surgical incision. The pyloric area should be located (this becomes easier with practice) or a portion of the omentum externalised for a better identification of anatomical structures. Next, select an area of the omentum that is not heavily vascularised to use as an attachment point (Fig. 15).

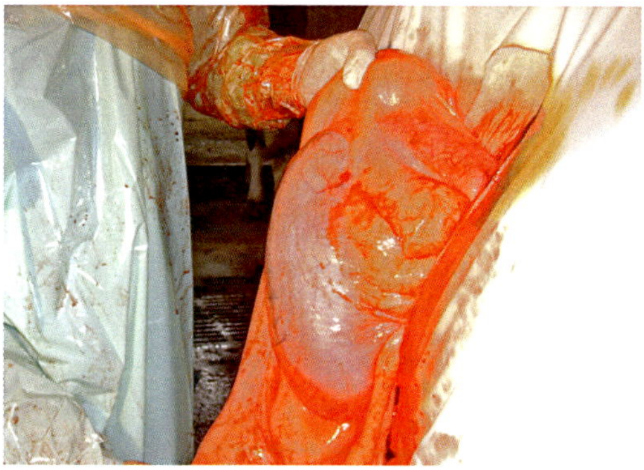

Figure 15. Abomasum externalised during surgery using the right flank approach. The most appropriate area for the suture is located next to the surgeon's thumb.

After choosing the most appropriate area of the omentum to which to attach the abomasum, the surgical technique to be used must be selected; this will vary depending on the surgeon and individual characteristics of the case. Regardless of the method chosen, the abomasum is attached to the abdominal wall, either independently or as part of the suture to close the muscular plane. The incision is then sutured, closing the wound layer by layer. Air should be removed from the abdomen; this requires an assistant to push on the ventral part of the abdomen on the left side while the surgeon sutures the layer that includes the peritoneum. The entry of air should also be avoided. Finally, the muscular, subcutaneous and cutaneous layers are sutured.

POSSIBLE DIFFICULTIES

If a large volume of gas is detected before attempting to correct the LDA, the viscera should be punctured with a needle connected to a tube. The needle and tubing will move with the abomasum during the repositioning of the latter. The procedure is continued as previously described for the right flank approach. In some cases, resolution can be quite complicated; e.g. if the animal has not been fasted in preparation for surgery, the abdomen will be particularly large due to the accumulation of rumen contents. Remember that cows with LDA can experience spontaneous transient changes in appetite.

Left flank approach

The procedures used for anaesthesia, surgical incision and closure are the same as those described for the right flank approach. The area should be prepared by shaving and disinfecting the right flank and the ventral region parallel to the linea alba.

Normally, the abomasum can be identified through the incision in the left flank (Fig. 16). After confirming the absence of adhesions, the omental region corresponding to the greater curvature of the abomasum is located. Here, a suture of about 150 cm in length is created using catgut or polyamide (USP 4 or 6) to attach the abomasum. Equal lengths of excess suture thread are left at the cranial and caudal ends of the suture (Fig. 17). Each of these ends is then externalised in an area of 5-10 cm parallel to and to the right of the linea alba and about 5-10 cm caudal to the xiphoid process.

In cows with a high body condition score, it is more difficult to handle the abomasum and omentum due to their increased weight and volume. Surgical intervention is easier in cows with a low body condition score, although the omental tissue can be scarce, increasing the likelihood of recurrence.

After lowering the abomasum by hand and removing the gas inside, the thread from the cranial side of the field is threaded through a Gerlarch needle (Fig. 18) and the abomasum is lowered cranially and ventrally (see explanation on p. 82). The advantages of the left flank approach are that the abomasum can be attached to abdominal floor and that the LDA

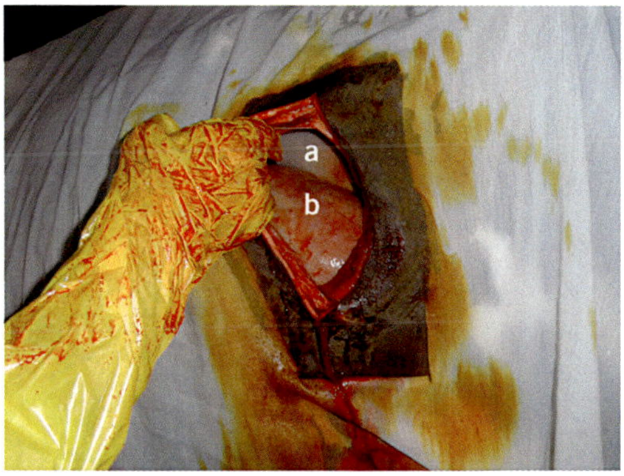

Figure 16. LDA surgery using the left flank approach. The rumen (a) and abomasum (b) are indicated.

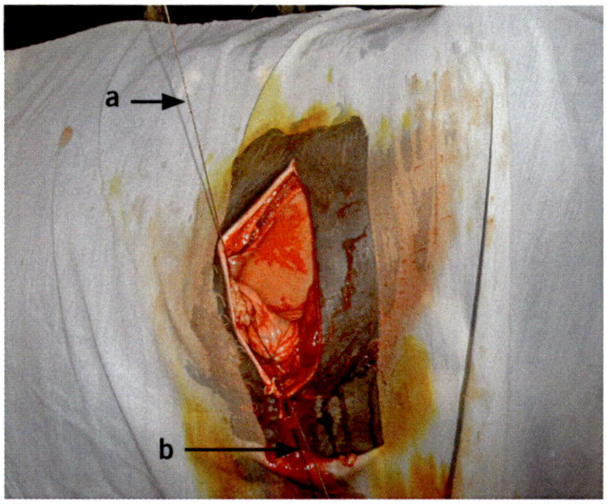

Figure 17. In the left flank approach, a poorly vascularised area of the omentum is used to attach the abomasum to the abdominal wall. Note the cranial (a) and caudal (b) ends of the suture thread, which is threaded though the Gerlach needle and used to attach the abomasum.

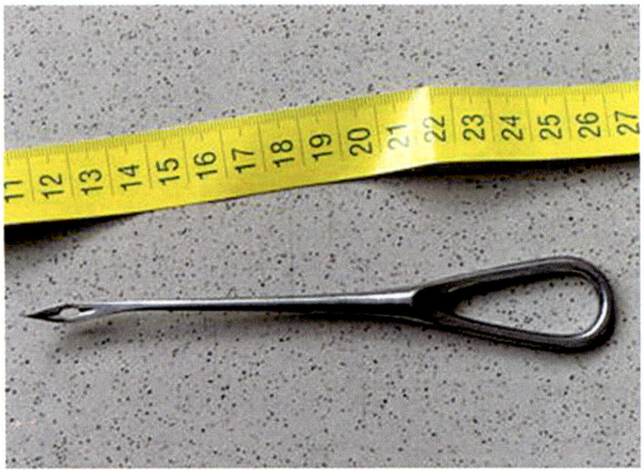

Figure 18. Gerlach needle.

rarely recurs. One drawback is that an assistant is required to remove the thread from the Gerlach needle. Moreover, the method can be very difficult if the animal has not been fasted beforehand.

Pharmacotherapy and monitoring

Regardless of the surgical approach chosen, post-operative drug treatment with antibiotics for 3 or 4 days and NSAIDs is required.

Recently operated cows need to be closely monitored for any signs of inflammation or possible complications of the surgical wound (see Case 3, p. 110). Diet should also be monitored and intake increased in the days after surgery. The cow should first be provided with rations containing good quality hay, and then gradually switched to a milking ration.

Mastitis

Mastitis is responsible for greater economic losses, both on farms and in the processing industry, than any other disease. One of the tasks of the cattle vet is to reduce a farm's costs during milk production. Accordingly, prevention of mastitis is especially important.

To obtain good quality milk and a good return on each farm, all milk quality management systems include critical control points and self-control systems. These systems are periodically audited, as this is the best way to control the production process and the final product.

PROCEDURE WITH GERLACH NEEDLE

Once the abomasum has been repositioned, and the ends of the suture thread brought to the outside of the incision, the needle is threaded and the first stitch is made with the help of an assistant, who indicates the correct location by pointing upwards from the outside with a blunt object, such as forceps. After fixing the abomasum in place, the Gerlach needle is brought to the outside of the incision and the thread removed from the needle. Next, the excess thread is used to create the first stitch with which to attach the abomasum to the abdominal wall. The surgeon then carefully removes the needle and repeats the procedure with the thread from the caudal end of the surgical field. Once the two ends of the thread have been adjusted from the outside, the surgeon should ensure that there is nothing between the omentum and peritoneum. Finally, the excess thread is knotted, leaving a long tail (about 10 cm) that is removed 7-12 days later.

However, in the absence of data on mastitis episodes on a given farm, it is difficult to accurately assess the problem, eliminate risk factors for a given outbreak and make the right decisions regarding the treatment or culling of the affected animals.

This section describes our experiences with bovine mastitis, and presents the results of a study conducted in collaboration with the University of Santiago de Compostela, Spain, and the Department of Agroforestry Engineering at the School of Engineering, in which the costs of mastitis on farms on the Spanish Cantabrian coast were estimated.

Estimated costs of mastitis

The aim of the study, titled "Estimating the costs of mastitis on dairy cattle farms" (Angel Castro, María Matilde Hernández and Jose Manuel Pereira), was to estimate the costs associated with mastitis on five dairy farms, considering the loss of production due three specific parameters: infection, treatment and milk discarded. This estimate did not include the costs of labour or veterinary care.

Compiled data

The data used in this study were collected between January 2008 and April 2009. We worked with various data pertaining to milk production and cell counts. Production and somatic cell counts (SCC) were monitored by monthly assessment of each individual cow. The cell counts obtained were transformed to a logarithmic scale (0-9), or linear score, which results in a normally distributed dataset, and thus simplifies the calculations and statistical analyses. The resulting values represent the SCC per cow per month, and can be used to predict the production losses per cow per day.

While records of mastitis treatment are generally not maintained on farms, these data were available from the certified dairy farms included in this study, and were recorded using a data sheet on which each of the following parameters was entered:

- Number or name of cow.
- Quarter affected (if applicable).
- Number of milkings during treatment.
- Number of milkings from which milk was discarded.
- Reason for treatment.
- Pharmacotherapy.
- Start and end dates of treatment and each dose administered.

This information complemented the production data and SCC of each animal. Although it is very important to keep track of all this information, this is rarely done on the majority of dairy farms.

Study results

In this study, data on the costs arising from cases of mastitis were collected during 2008 and the first quarter of 2009, while data on the costs per cow were collected only in 2008. The latter reflects the cost assumed per lactating cow; i.e. the cost of mastitis divided by the total number

PRODUCTION LOSSES

Production losses associated with different SCC values are determined by considering the linear score (LS) and the loss of milk/cow/day:
(LS - 2) x 0.66

All cows with a SCC > 200,000 cells/ml were evaluated.

of cows on the farm, and not just those affected by mastitis.

Costs of discarded milk

Table 2 shows the costs per cow and per case of mastitis due to milk that could not be sold due to non-compliance with the treatment withdrawal period.

- The quantity of milk discarded due to mastitis ranged from 198.5 to 299 kg/case (mean: 231.8 kg). These figures translated to a mean loss of €80 per case* (range: €69.40 to €105.50).
- The mean amount of milk discarded per lactating cow on each farm was 228.8 kg/cow/year or €82.50/cow/year (range: €24.50 to €161.60/cow/year).

Treatment costs

Table 3 shows the treatment cost per cow per case of mastitis.

- The mean cost per case was €116.30 (range: €75.80 to €172.50).
- The mean cost was €37.40/cow/year (range: €13 to €74.50/cow/year).

Costs due to loss of production

The largest mean production losses were incurred in June and July. These losses varied widely, ranging from 500 L to over 4,500 L of milk per month, depending on the size of the herd.

Table 2. Cost of milk discarded per cow and per case of mastitis.

Farm	1	2	3	4	5	Mean
Cost per case						
Unsold milk kg/case	220	214.9	198.5	226.6	299.1	**231.8**
€/case	74.5	73.8	69.4	77.6	105.5	**80.2**
Cost per cow (determined for all cows in the herd, with and without mastitis)						
Unsold milk kg/cow/year	72.9	449.5	69.7	344.8	207	**228.8**
€/cow/year	25.9	161.6	24.5	124.9	75.5	**82.5**

* The cost of losses was calculated based on the price of milk in the years during which the study was conducted (2008-2009).

Table 3. Costs of treatments administered per cow and per case of mastitis.

Farm	1	2	3	4	5	Mean
Coste per case						
€/case	156.2	86.8	75.8	172.5	90.1	**116.3**
Cost per cow						
€/cow/year	28.3	74.5	13	36.6	34.6	**37.4**

Table 4. Costs of lost production per cow.

Farm	1	2	3	4	5	Mean
Cost per cow						
Cost of unsold milk per cow (kg/cow)	299	249.3	295.5	266.4	265.4	**275.1**
€/cow/year	110.5	91.3	108.7	97.6	98.1	**101.2**

Table 4 shows the cost per cow per year due to lost production caused by subclinical mastitis.

The mean production loss was 275.1 kg/cow/year, although this cost varies from 249.3 to 299 kg/cow/year. This translates to a mean cost of €101.2 / cow/year (range: €91.3 to €110.5/cow/year).

Table 4 does not include the estimated cost per case of mastitis, as no data were available on specific SSC values for each treatment, which would have allowed us to determine the decrease in production due to each individual case of mastitis. Regardless, total costs due to the loss of milk production, calculated for all recorded cases of mastitis, were estimated at an average of €145 per case. Although these calculations do not exactly reflect reality, as production losses were calculated for the entire herd, they provide a useful indication of the cost of subclinical mastitis, which usually goes unnoticed and untreated.

Conclusion

Adding together the three costs studied (milk discarded, treatment and loss of production) gives an average cost per cow per year of €221.10. Of this amount, 46 % was due to production loss (in agreement with Mintelburg, 2007), 37 % to discarded milk, and 17 % to treatment costs.

The average cost per case of mastitis was €196; this was calculated by considering only the cost of discarded milk and the cost of treatment, with the latter accounting for up to 59 % of the final estimate.

Ultimately, the costs associated with mastitis are very high. The graph in Figure 19 summarises the losses incurred on the farms studied throughout 2008. The average amount lost by each of these farms was €13,863, although this ranged from €5,950 to €14,650 on individual farms.

Figure 19. Graph summarising losses per farm.

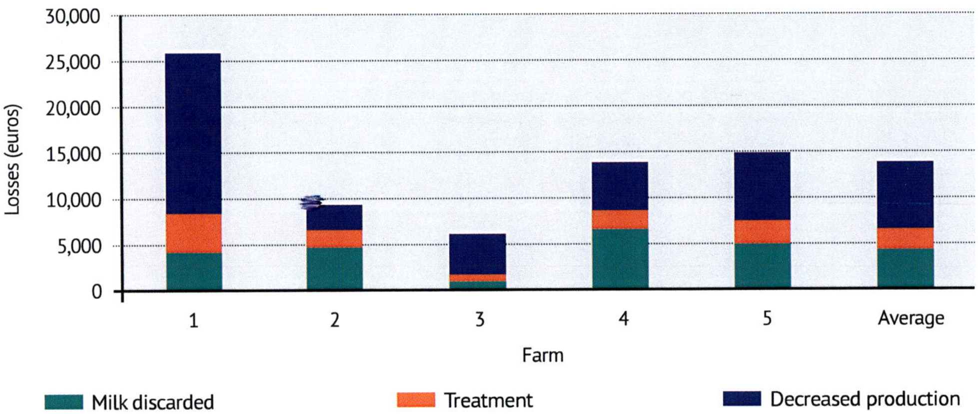

6

General management

The management of cattle is a subject so vast that an entire publication could be easily devoted to this topic. In this chapter, we will focus on issues related to the peripartum period that directly result in an imbalance in the cascade of metabolic changes that occurs at this time. Any management decisions that affect the animal's welfare can trigger this imbalance.

Collective management

In general terms, good management seeks to ensure adequate animal welfare during all of the cow's activities:

- Feeding.
- Drinking.
- Resting.
- Exercising.

Solid feed

Cows should be provided with sufficient amounts of good quality feed.

Amount

On some farms, rations are prepared to feed animals for two days; this is not a major problem as long as the weather is not too hot and the feed is always accessible to the cows (Fig. 1). However, problems can arise if the ration contains unstable ingredients. In any case, feed palatability is always worse when distributed as a single ration. Fresh cows are the most sensitive to changes in feeding routines.

Feed should be available practically 24 hours per day.

The system of food distribution should be altered if animals are found to lack feed at certain times (Fig. 2).

Quality

As regards feed quality, the microbiological and nutritional aspects of feed should be considered. The farm's nutritionist should ensure that animals are provided with an appropriate, balanced ration, which should be correctly distributed (Figs. 3-8).

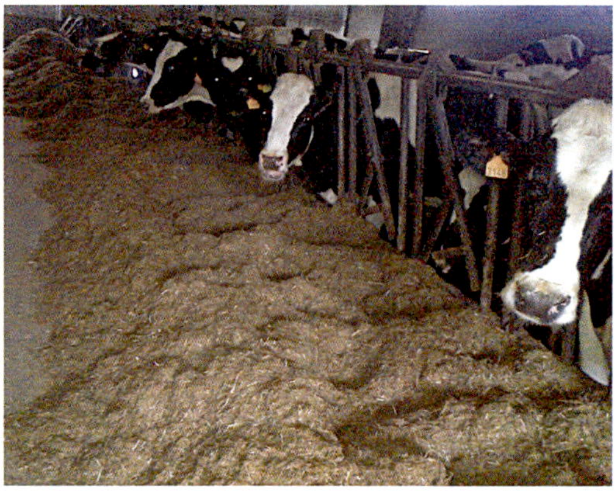

Figure 1. Two-day ration distributed with the Unifeed system.

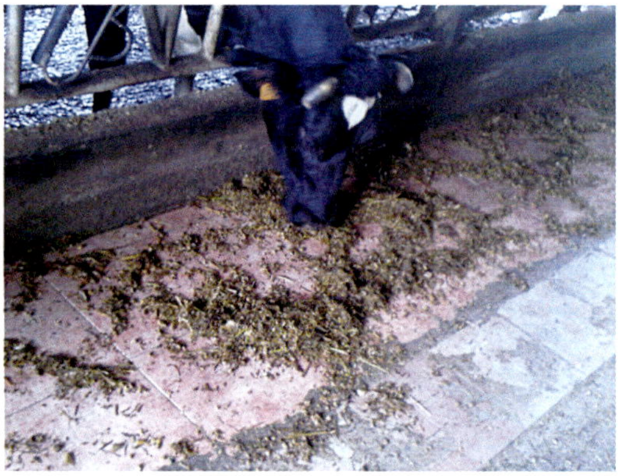

Figure 2. Feeding table containing little feed.

SOLID FEED

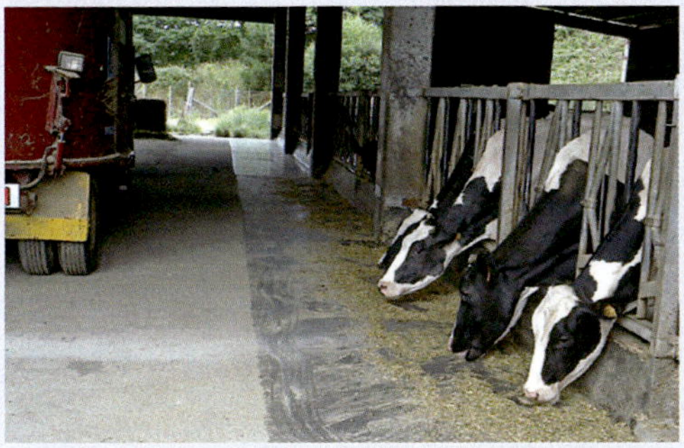

Figure 3. Ration distributed over a smooth, easily cleaned, resin surface. Stainless steel surfaces are a good economic alternative.

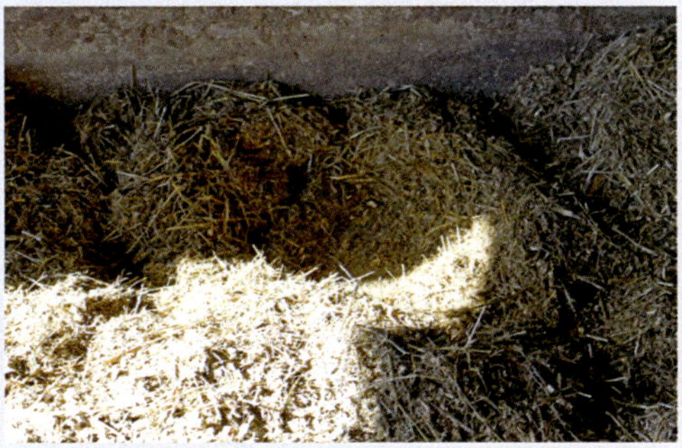

Figure 4. Avoid exposing feed to direct light and heat for a long time.

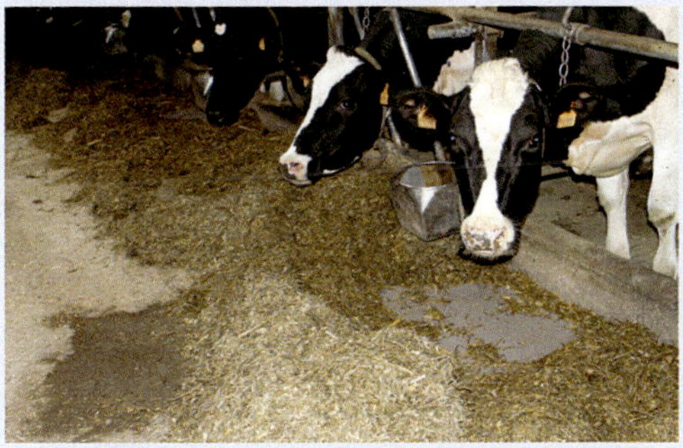

Figure 5. It is more difficult to detect cows that are not feeding when using a Unifeed system for food distribution, as compared with a fixed position system in which the cow does not move and feed build-up can be easily observed. In this case, the second cow from the right is not feeding well.

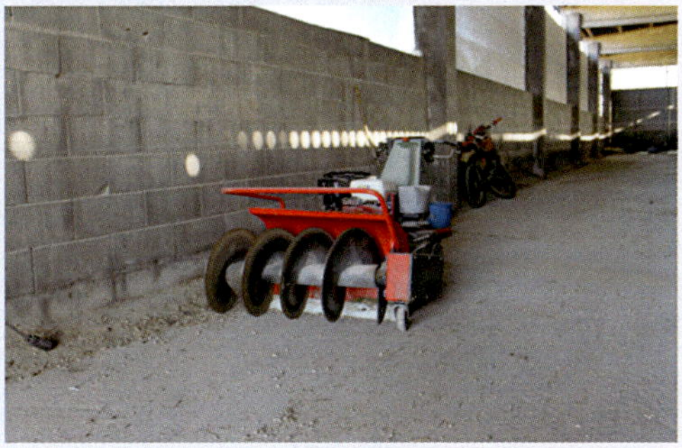

Figure 6. Automated feed pusher in the feeding area so feed can be more easily accessed by the cows.

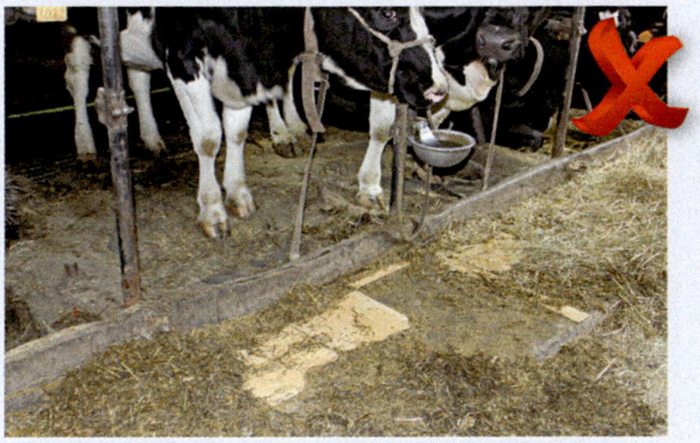

Figure 7. Tiled feeding table in poor condition.

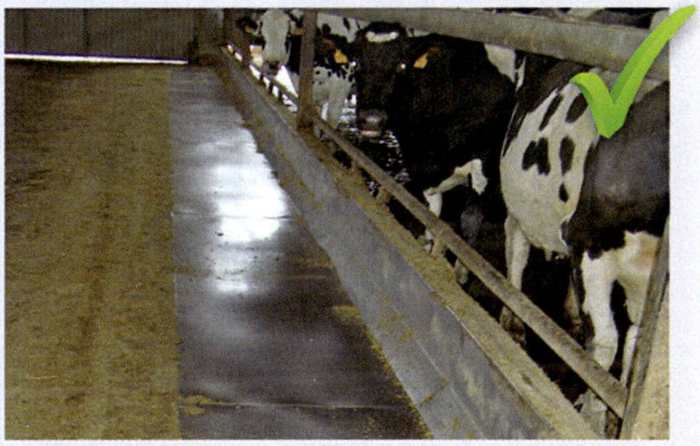

Figure 8. Good condition, easily cleaned, metal feeding surface.

Water should be available almost 24 hours a day.

Water intake

Good quality water should be available in sufficient quantities. Drinking water must meet certain hygienic and organoleptic requirements, and should always be freely available to the animals (Fig. 9). The use of chlorine dispensers or other water purification products is highly recommended to ensure good water quality at all times. The investment necessary to acquire this type of water purification system is minimal compared to the long-term benefits (Figs. 10-13).

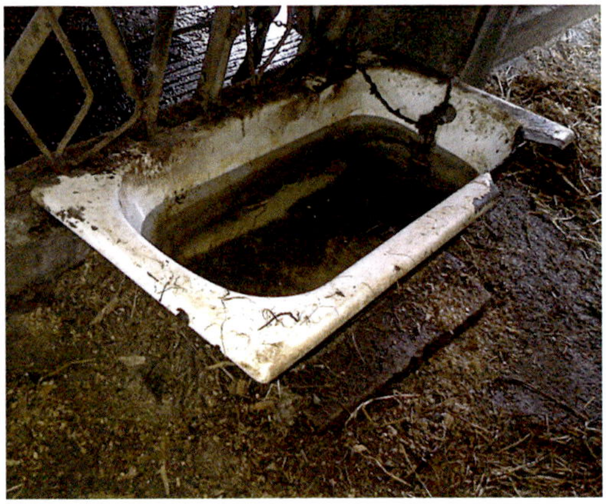

Figure 9. Dirty drinking trough with sharp, potentially dangerous corners.

WATER INTAKE

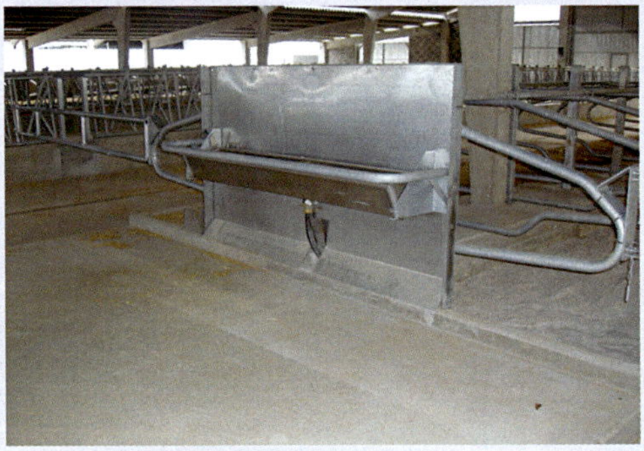

Figure 10. Drinking troughs should be accessible and contain sufficient amounts of good quality water.

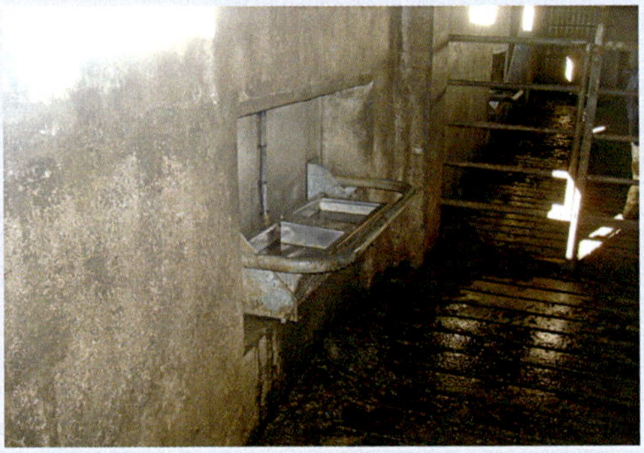

Figure 11. If the troughs are not easily accessible, they should at least be protected so as to avoid any accidents.

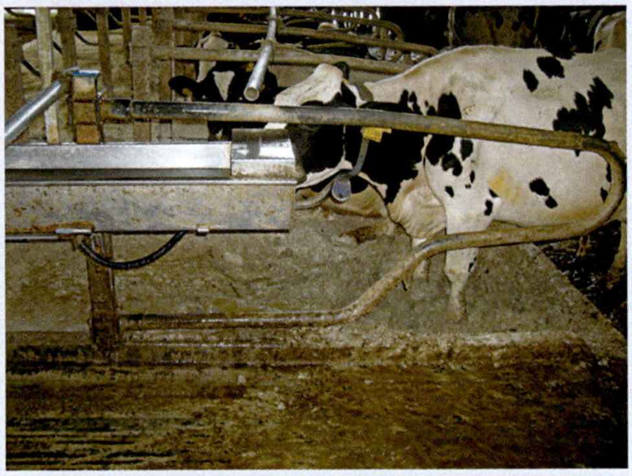

Figure 12. In this case, the location of the trough causes drinking cows to spill water, which floods the adjacent cubicle.

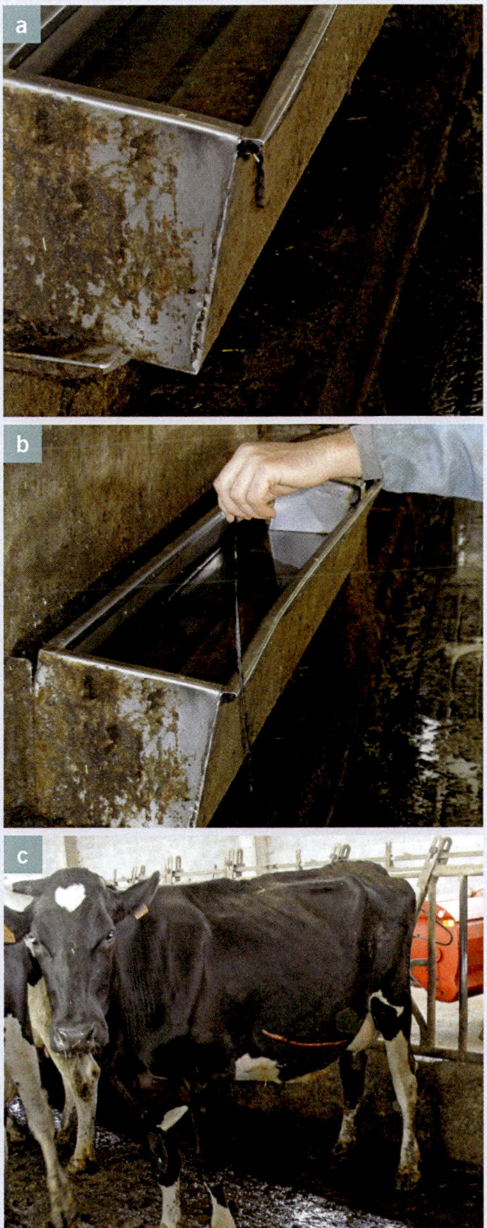

Figure 13. Drinking troughs with protrusions may cause accidents (a). The edges of the trough can catch the cow and cause tears in the skin (b). Note the injury caused by the drinking trough to the cow pictured above (c).

Rest

The design and layout of the cubicles in which cows are housed is of fundamental importance for the welfare of the animals (Fig. 14). Neil Anderson outlines the six most important requirements that a cubicle must fulfil for the animals to rest properly:

- Enough space to lie on either flank, with unobstructed space for the neck and head.
- Enough space to rest the head against either side while standing (without obstruction by the cubicle divider bars).
- Enough space for cows to lie down and rest their legs, udders and tails on a horizontal surface.
- Enough space to stand or lie down without being injured by neck rails, partitions, or supports.
- A clean, dry soft bed.

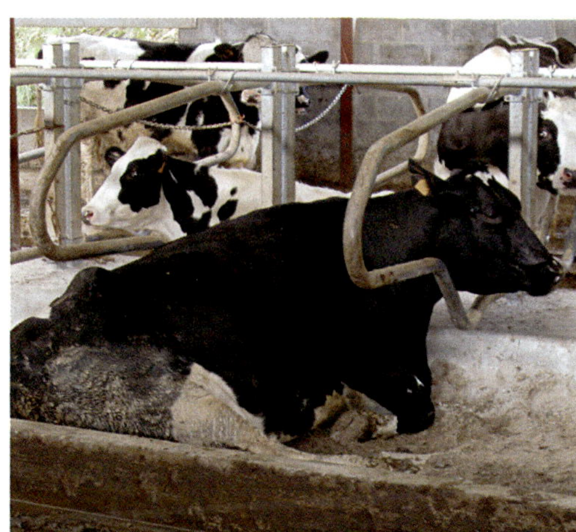

Figure 14. Cow resting properly. Note that the cow has enough space in the cubicle to move its head to either side.

In addition to these six basic requirements, the following recommendations regarding the occupancy rate of the cubicles in the stalls should also be adhered to:

- Dry cow batch: 90 % occupancy.
- Prepartum batch: 85 % occupancy and slightly wider beds.

The cleanliness of the facilities also influences the health and welfare of animals (Figs. 15-21).

If the facilities in which the cows are housed are suitably hygienic, exposure to pollutants and infectious agents will be decreased.

TYPES OF REST CUBICLES

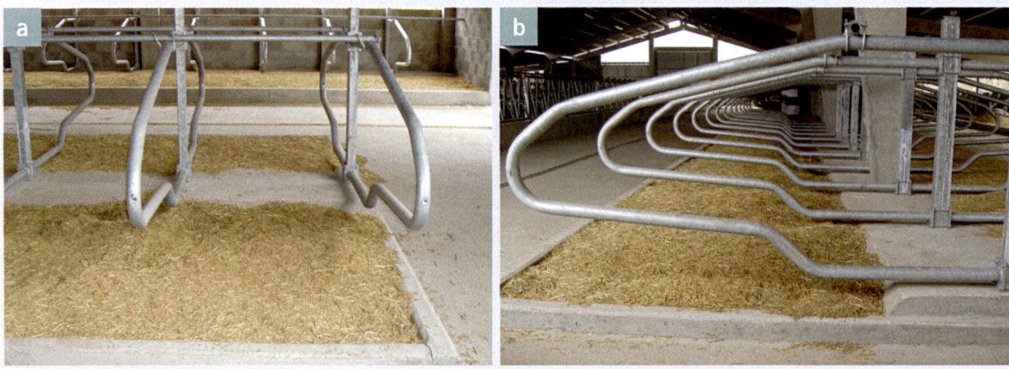

Figure 15. Well-designed cubicle; front (a) and side (b) views.

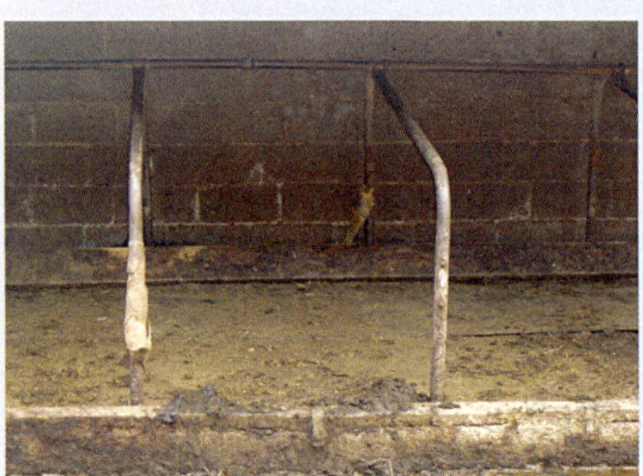

Figure 16. Poorly designed cubicle.

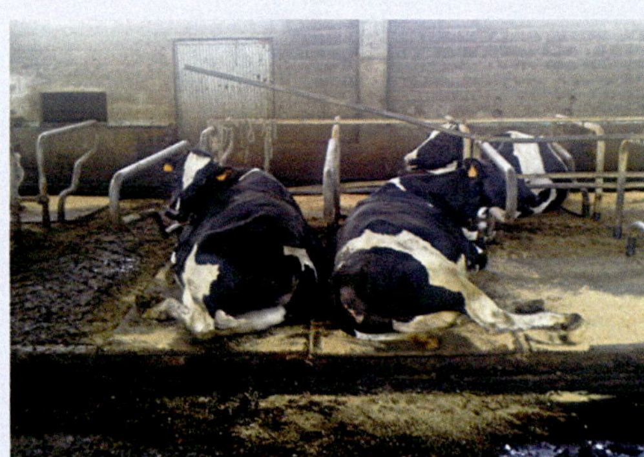

Figure 17. Properly designed but poorly maintained cubicles.

Figure 22 shows a facility in which the automatic cleaning system is broken and does not fully clean the aisle. The area closest to the bed remains dirty and the rear of the cow (i.e. vagina, tail, udder, etc.), which should be kept clean, is exposed to excrement.

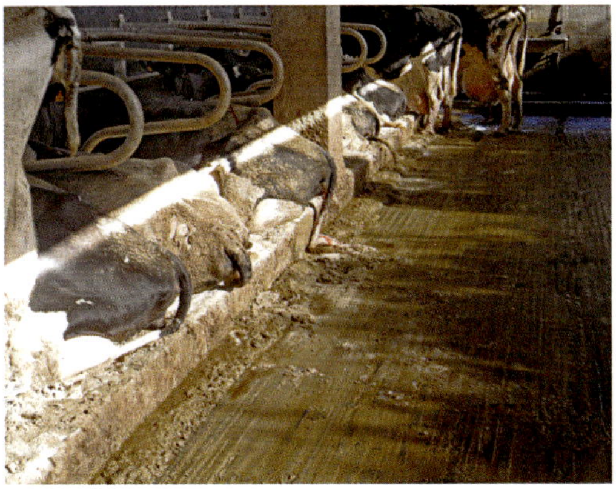

Figure 22. A failure of the automatic cleaning system results in the accumulation of organic residues near the beds.

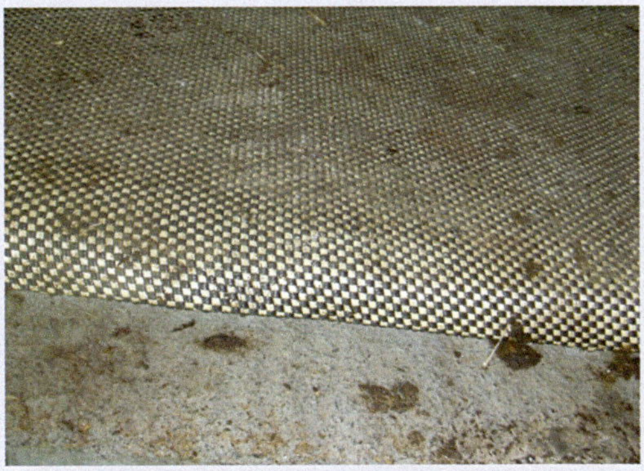

Figure 18. Beds should be comfortable and flat. The bed shown in the photograph should be covered with a layer of sand or other material.

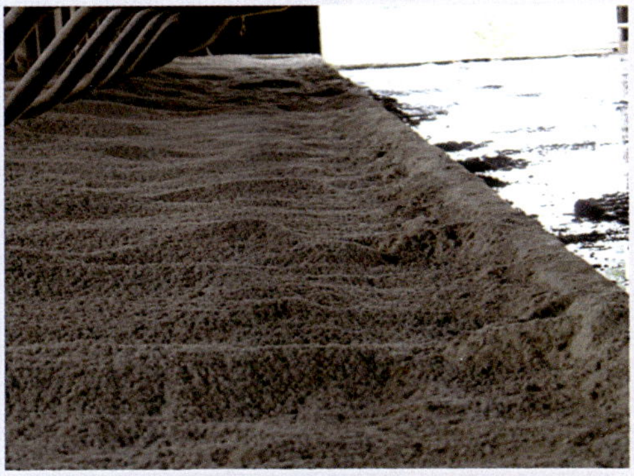

Figure 19. A good sand bedding provides a comfortable, easy to clean surface.

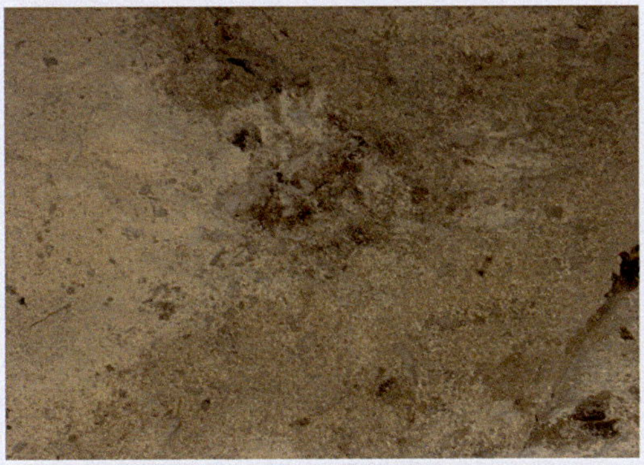

Figure 20. Note the accumulation of dirt on the bed. Regular maintenance and cleaning of the beds is essential to prevent mastitis.

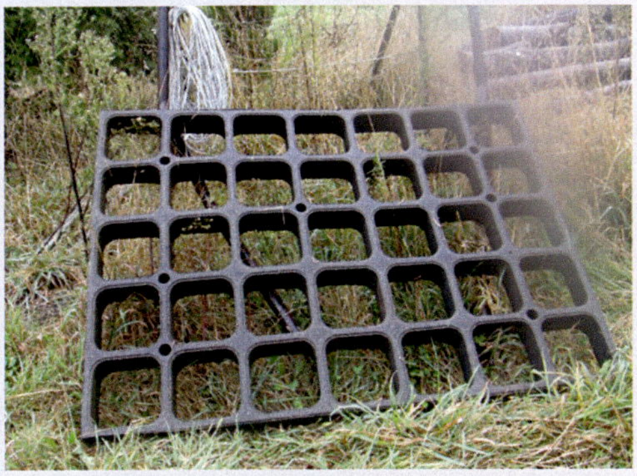

Figure 21. Rubber matting, which limits the amount of bedding used, provides a useful base on which to spread the bedding material.

Cubicle dimensions

Figure 23 shows the appropriate steps for designing a rest cubicle for a cow.

Poorly designed cubicles on a cattle farm can result in the following situations:

1. Cows attempt to adapt their position to fit inside the cubicle (perching between the cubicle and the aisle) (Fig. 24).
2. The consequence of perching is that most of the animals remain standing, unsure of whether to stand or lie down.

The following behaviours may indicate that the dimensions of the cubicle do not allow the cow to rest comfortably:

- Sniffing the ground for some time before making any movement.
- Repeatedly moving head from side to side due to a lack of sufficient space.
- Making numerous attempts before lying down or standing up (Fig. 25).

This kind of discomfort can result in poor posture, although this problem can usually be easily

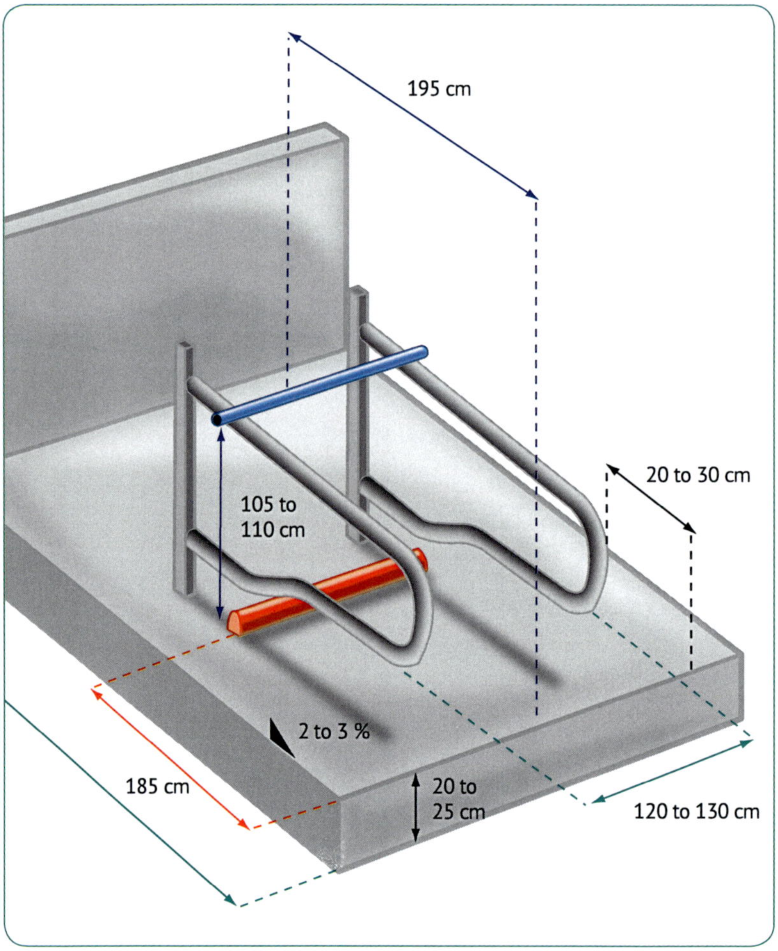

Figure 23. Diagram showing the appropriate measurements of a rest cubicle for a cow. Adapted from Colleu, B. «Le gabarit des vaches évolue, le réglage des logettes aussi». PLM. *Production laitière moderne*, June 2009, p. 30-32.

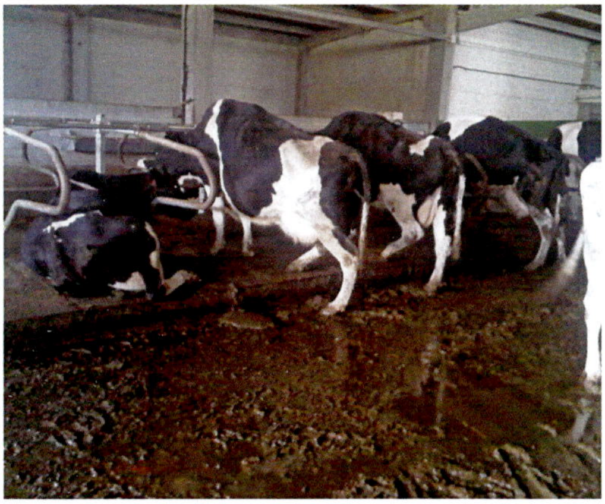

Figure 24. Cows standing with the front feet in the cubicle and the rear feet in the aisle (perching). They remain unsure of whether to stand or lie down for long periods of time.

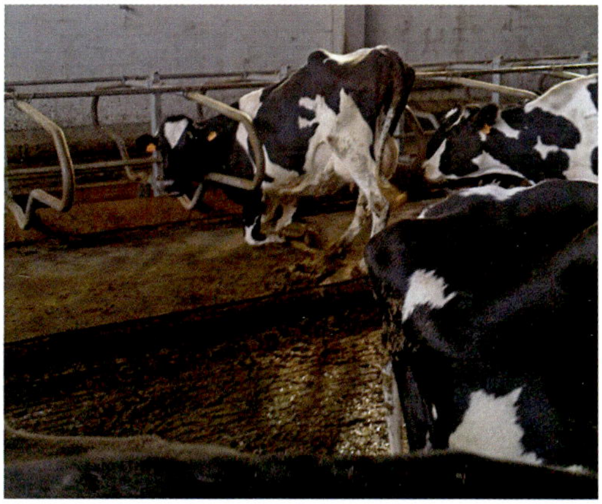

Figure 25. As it attempts to lie down, the cow repeatedly kneels down and stands up.

solved. Figure 26 shows a cow with poor posture. Note that the cow is prevented from moving forward by the upper horizontal bar of the cubicle, which is about 40 cm from the wall, as well as by the lower bar. This cubicle design makes it difficult for the cow to comfortably lie down, and gives rise to postural problems. Normally, after eating, 85 % of the animals should be lying in the cubicles. Of these 50 % of should be ruminating. Two hours later, 90 % of the group should be lying in the cubicles (Fig. 27). If these figures are not observed, it suggests a problem that prevents the cows from lying down (Figs. 28-34).

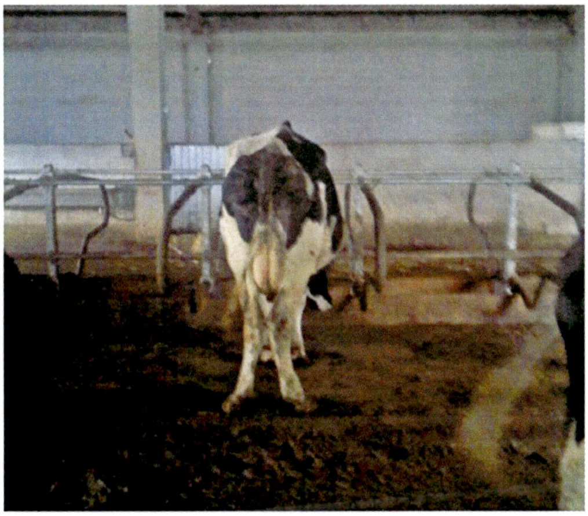

Figure 26. Cow with bad posture in a poorly designed cubicle.

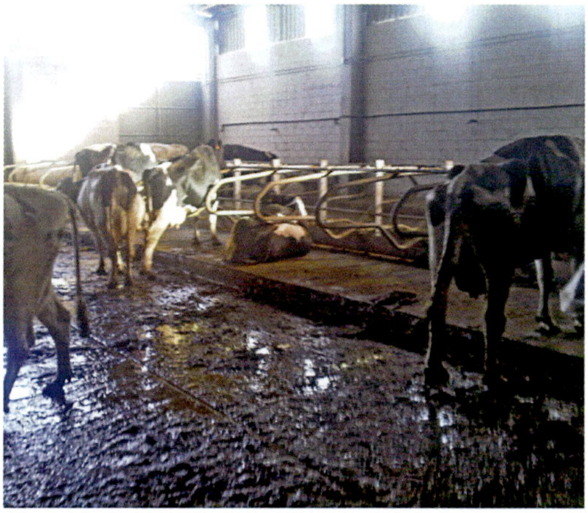

Figure 27. Many cows standing, regardless of the time of day, is indicative of a problem in the design of the cubicles.

REST FACILITIES AND CUBICLES

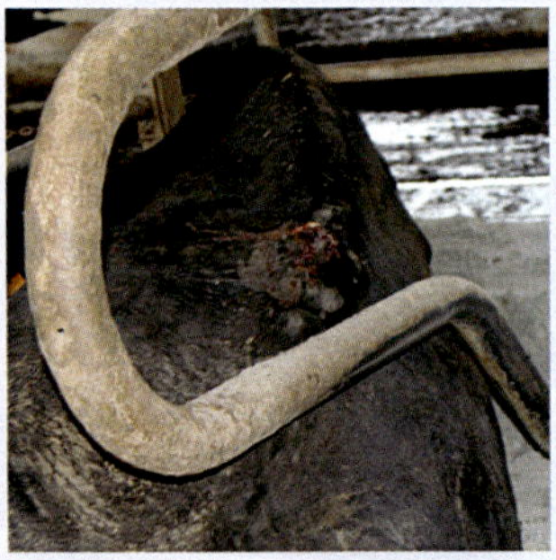

Figure 28. Bad cubicle design results in repeated injuries to the back of the cow. In this case, the problem is exaggerated because the cow is lame. This cow should be moved to another location.

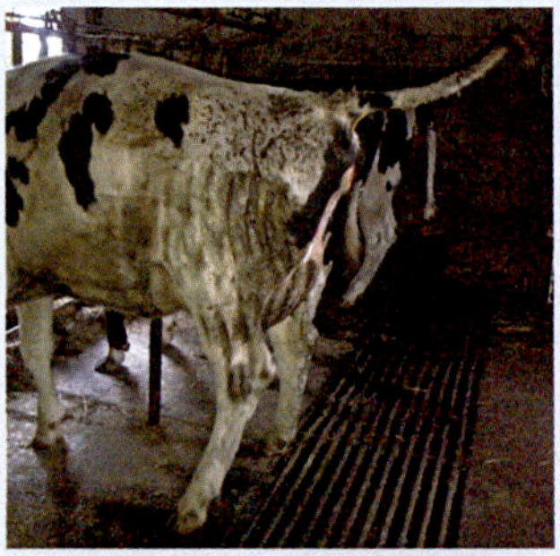

Figure 29. In a fixed stabling system with a grill, cows can end up resting directly on the grill if the beds are not appropriately sized. Note the marks on the cow's hindlimb, which suggest that the animal is not comfortable.

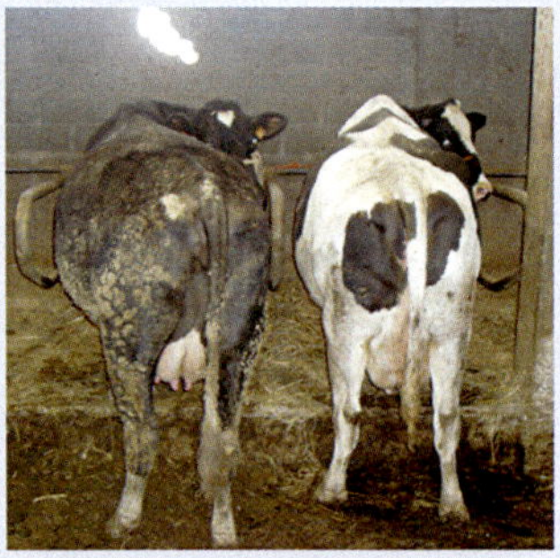

Figure 30. Cows should be relatively clean. When the design and cleaning of cubicles are inadequate, cows can be observed with some areas of the body clean and others dirty.

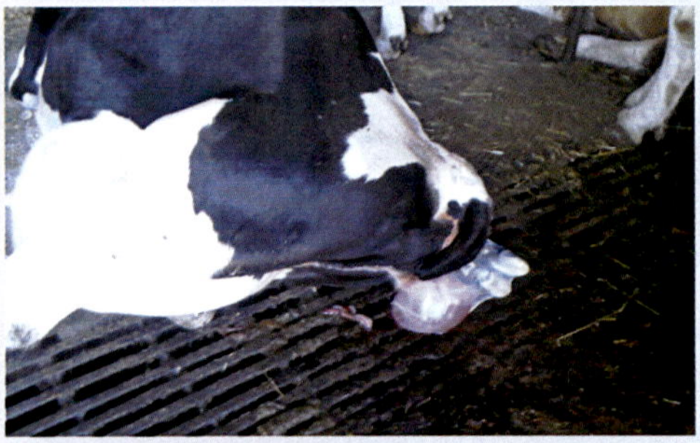

Figure 31. A grill contaminated with faeces is not the best place to calve.

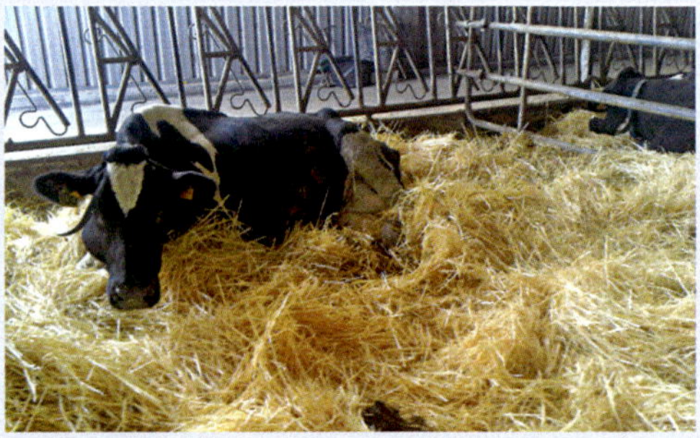

Figure 32. Delivery areas should be spacious and clean.

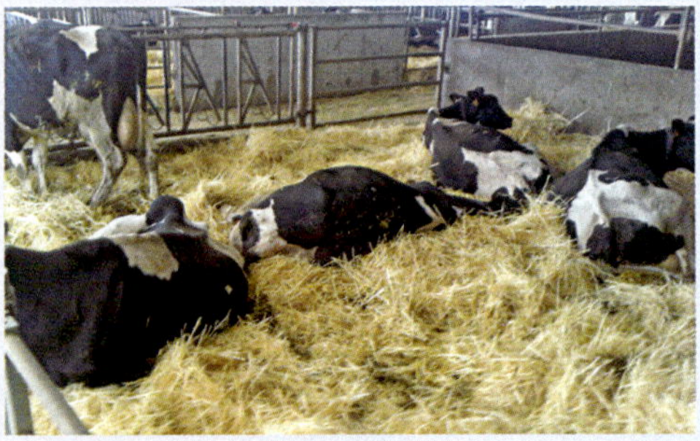

Figure 33. Fresh cows should be housed in comfortable and uncrowded facilities.

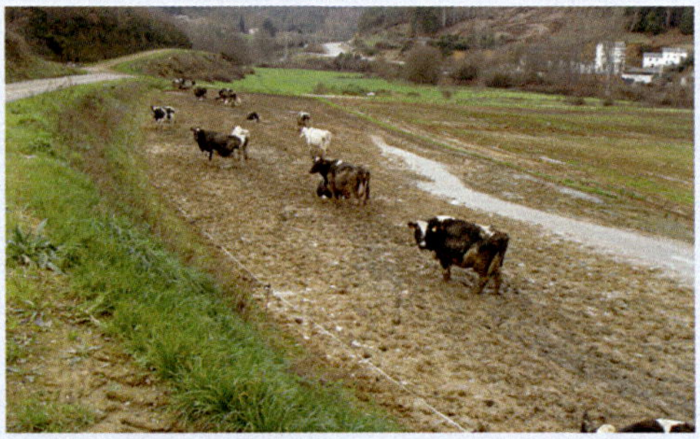

Figure 34. On many farms, dry cows are often kept outside in inappropriate areas.

Exercise

Exercise is important for pregnant cows, which should be provided with adequate space. Cows that have recently calved, and hence been exposed to significant stress, should resume regular physical activity (Figs. 35-46).

ANIMAL COMFORT (I)

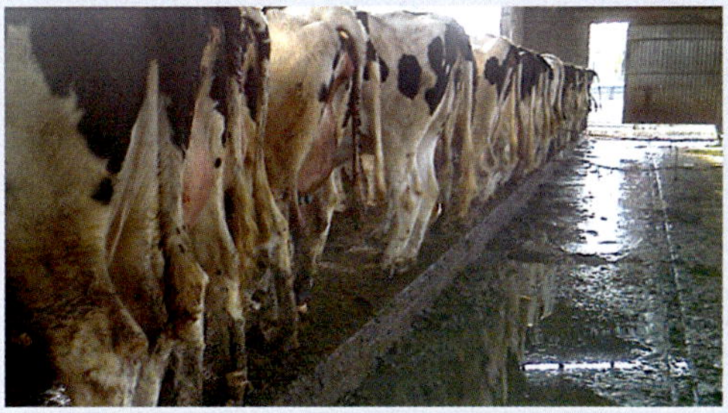

Figure 35. The position of the animals in the feeding area is sometimes conditioned by the presence of steep steps, which can cause leg injuries.

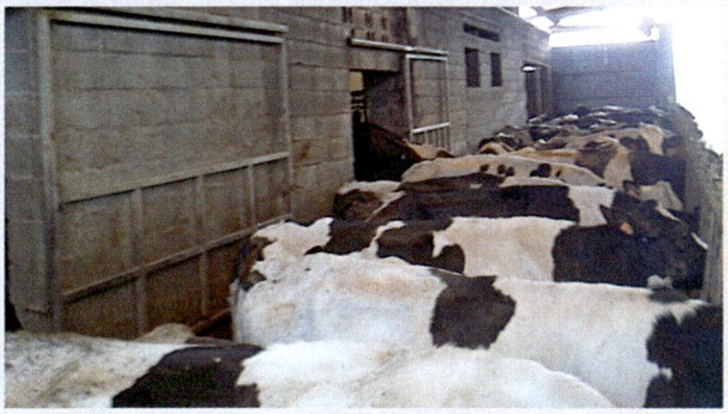

Figure 36. The aisles of the facilities must be sufficiently wide.

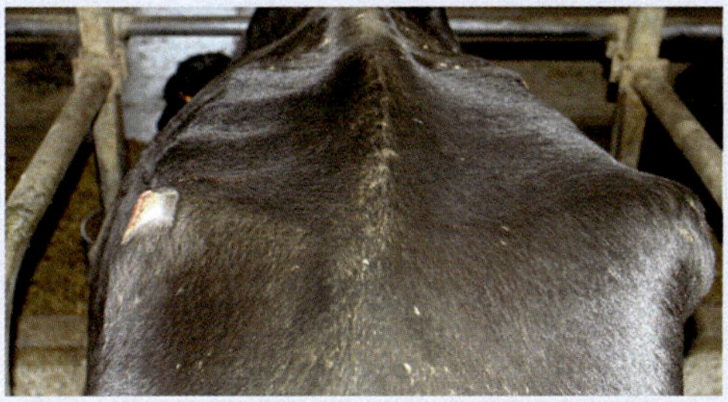

Figure 37. The corridors or entrance or exit doors must be free of bottlenecks or protrusions that are likely to cause injury.

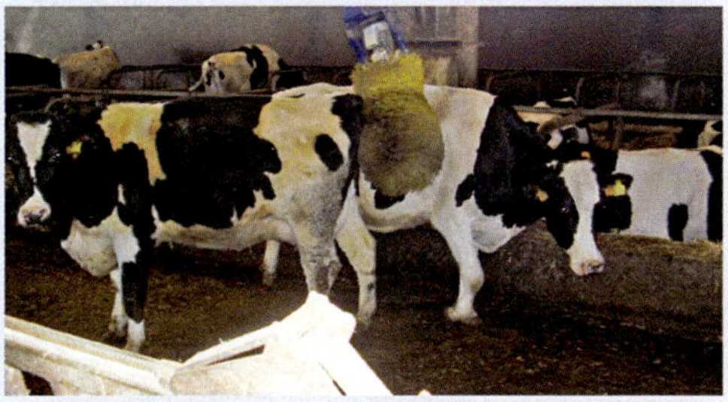

Figure 38. Cleaning brushes, which can have anti-stress effects, can improve the comfort and welfare of cows.

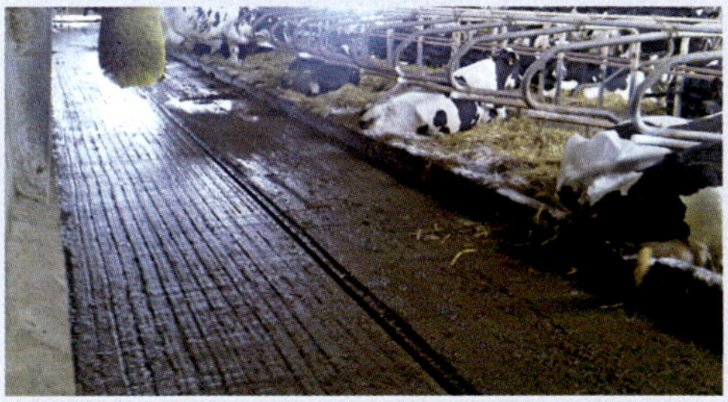

Figure 39. Comfortable supportive surfaces, such as rubber mats in the hallways, should be provided.

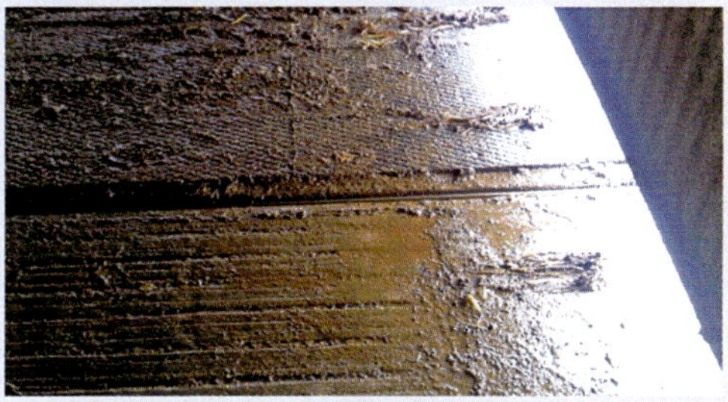

Figure 40. On this farm, half the aisle has been covered with rubber matting.

ANIMAL COMFORT (II)

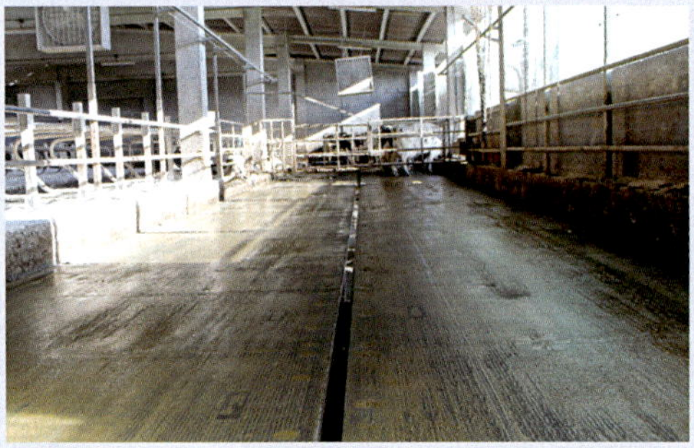

Figure 41. Farm in which the entire aisle has been covered with rubber matting.

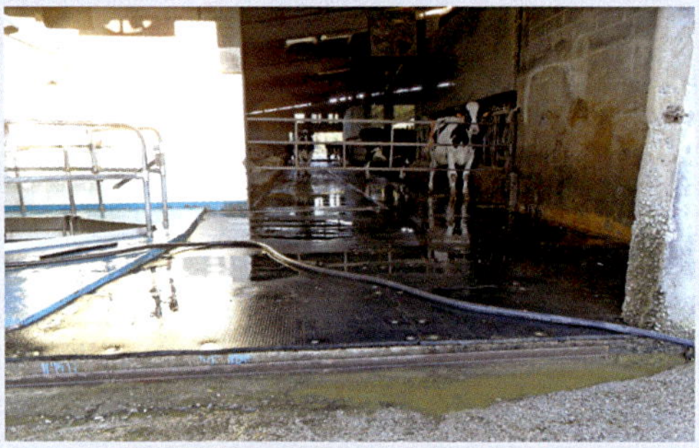

Figure 42. Note the matting in the waiting area. This greatly enhances the comfort of the animals, especially on farms that perform three milkings per day, which requires that the cows be held in this area for long periods of time.

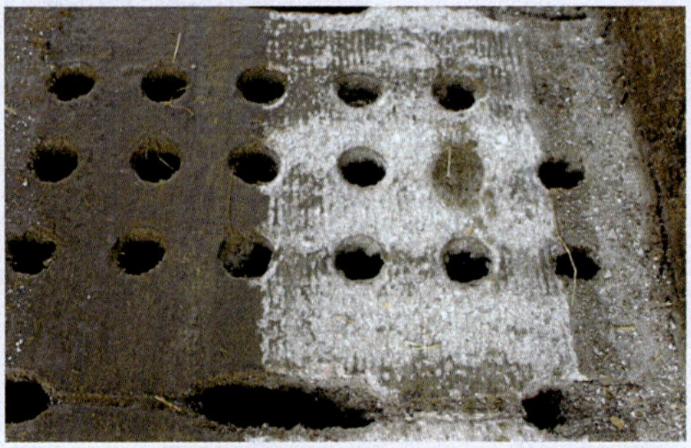

Figure 43. Care should be taken to ensure that the floor does not become slippery. On this farm, grooves have been carved in the concrete (white part, right).

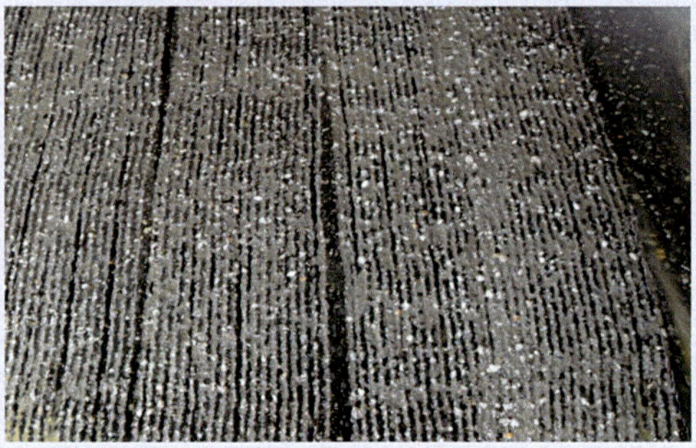

Figure 44. Note the fully grooved floor on this farm.

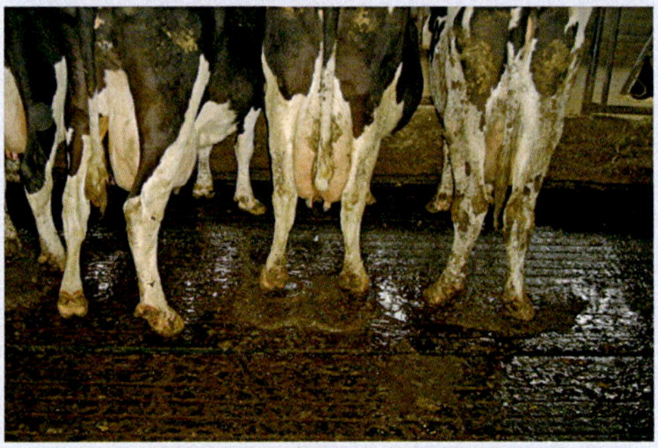

Figure 45. The stance (foot angle) helps to indicate the degree of comfort of the animals. The frequency with which the hooves are trimmed should be recorded.

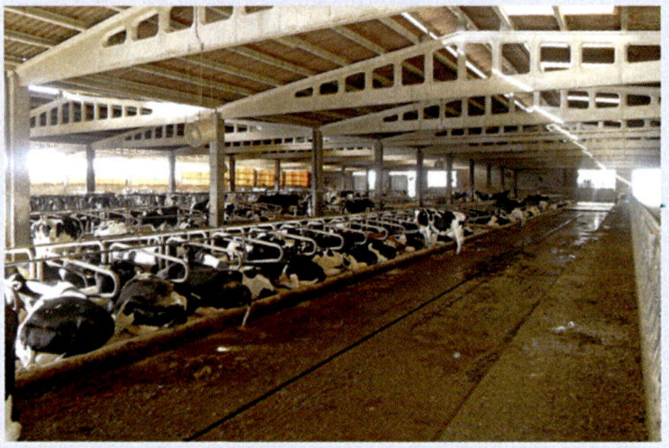

Figure 46. If most of the cows are resting (up to 90 % lying down two hours after eating), the facilities are suitably comfortable.

Individual management

During the peripartum period, cows require specific management strategies according to their particular situation.

In first-lactation cows, a minimum of 45 days of drying is recommended to ensure good future production.

Planning the dry period

Table 1 shows data for dry cows on a farm. In this example, there are eight dry cows and the farmer has predicted a mean dry period of 82 days from the expected calving date; this exceeds the recommended 60 days. The adult cows are those with the greatest deviation from the estimated dry period length.

By analysing these data, we can identify cows with a high risk of metabolic problems and take the appropriate action in time.

- The duration of the dry period of cows 4, 5, 6 and 7 is too long. This is due to several factors: they have taken too long to become pregnant, and have had to be dried off very early due to production problems, mastitis, etc.
- The dry period of cow 1 is too short; this happens to be a first-calf cow. Data like these are typically obtained for cows that are good producers, and for which the drying-off date is delayed on purpose. This practice is especially discouraged in heifers.

Table 2 shows another analysis of the data from Table 1.

Table 1. Dry cow data. Source: cowsulting.com

Cow	Calving number	Expected dry-off date (60 days)	Actual dry-off date	Deviation in dry-off date (days)	Expected calving date*	Actual duration of dry period
1	1	24/09/2012	18/10/2012	24	23/11/2012	36
2	1	11/11/2012	13/11/2012	2	10/01/2013	58
3	2	06/09/2012	05/09/2012	-1	05/11/2012	61
4	4	11/10/2012	12/09/2012	-29	10/12/2012	89
5	5	15/09/2012	17/07/2012	-60	14/11/2012	120
6	6	07/10/2012	12/09/2012	-25	06/12/2012	85
7	7	30/11/2012	05/09/2012	-86	29/01/2013	146
8	9	11/11/2012	13/11/2012	2	10/01/2013	58

*In practice, if calving is delayed, the number of estimated days of drying is altered.

Table 2. Dry cow summary data. Source: www.cowsulting.com

Dry period	Number of cows	Dry days (mean)	< 40 days	40-70 days	> 70 days
1st calving	2	47	1	1	0
2nd calving	1	61	0	1	0
≥ 3rd calving	5	100	0	1	4
Total	8	82	1	3	4

Twin pregnancy

In cases of twin pregnancies, delivery should be expected earlier than the estimated calving date. The difference between the actual and estimated calving dates depends on the characteristics of the foetus; for example, calving is delayed in cases in which calves are sired by a beef bull. These parameters must be taken into account when planning the drying-off date in order to avoid problems.

The most common postpartum diseases in cases of twin pregnancy are: hypocalcaemia, retained placenta and displaced abomasum. Thus, cows that are pregnant with twins should be monitored, and before calving the calving number and any deficiencies shown by the mother should be noted. Some of the preventative measures that can be taken include restorative therapy with calcium, oxytocin or ergonovine (if applicable) and housing the cow in a large space (which favours calving); these females need more space and greater comfort.

REMEMBER

After calving twins, a large space is freed up in the abdomen, and thus these cows are at greater risk of abomasal displacement. Monitor the animal!

Heifers

For obvious reasons, heifers require a longer period of adaptation for each of the phases of their first calving. This event constitutes the first major stress to which these cows are exposed. Generally, heifers require twice as much time as adult cows to adapt to a new diet, although this depends on the previous diet and that to which they are being introduced (Fig. 47).

In some places (such as the Cantabrian coast, in the north of Spain), heifers often remain at pasture before calving, where they are less closely monitored. Accordingly, these cows should be managed carefully, especially in cases involving poor development or body condition.

Heifers remain in the growth phase after their first calving, resulting in a lower yield per animal and a lower body condition score.

Grazing cows

Cows that are kept at pasture during the dry period will be less closely monitored than stabled animals (Fig. 48). Moreover, grazing cows often do not have access to the minerals necessary to fulfil their nutritional requirements. Cows grazing on fresh grass are also at greater risk of hypocalcaemia due to alterations in the metabolic anion/cation balance caused by the high calcium content of grass. This situation should be prevented.

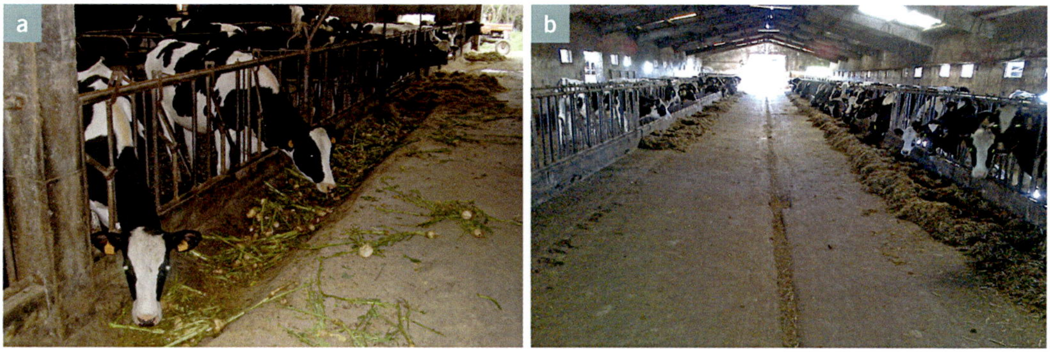

Figure 47. The feed and rations provided to heifers should be in accordance with the nutritionist's recommendations, and should not be decided upon by the farmer on a whim.

From a nutritional standpoint, it is preferable to stable the cows during the prepartum period; this allows closer monitoring and a more progressive transition to the postpartum diet. However, it should be borne in mind that stabling cows that were previously kept at pasture involves a change in the batch, which itself causes a certain degree of stress.

Cows should ideally have access to feed supplements during the prepartum and dry periods.

Batch creation and movement

Movements should be carefully planned; the less the cows are moved, the better. The ideal solution is to house dry cows and heifers using a freestall system. If heifers cannot be kept inside, they should be familiarised with the cubicles one or two months before calving to allow for adaptation. It is also recommended to drive the cows through the milking parlour so that they become accustomed to the narrow aisles.

Ideally, postpartum heifers should be separated from the postpartum batch, although in practice this is not always possible. Grouping heifers and adult cows in the same batch can trigger hierarchical problems and postpartum diseases (see Case 4, p. 114) (Figs. 49-53).

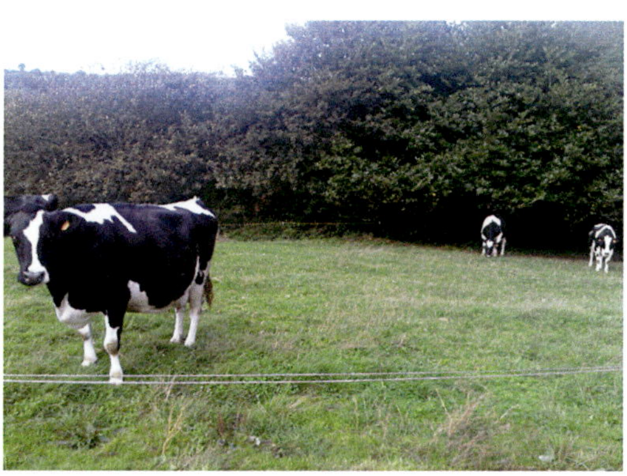

Figure 48. Dry cows kept at pasture.

Animals should always be moved in groups in order to minimise stress.

Prevention of postpartum metabolic problems in dry cows

Chapter 5 provides more detail on the range of postpartum diseases. In general, however, pre- and postpartum prevention protocols should be adhered to in order to avoid these problems. It is especially important to apply these measures

BATCH CREATION AND MOVEMENT

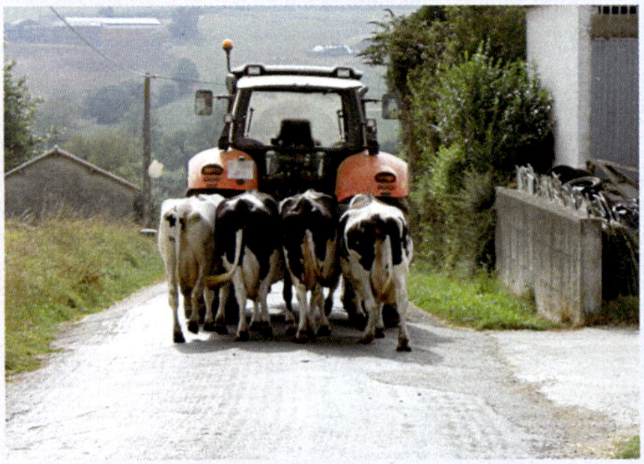

Figure 49. Moving dry cows to pasture can constitute a sudden change for the animals concerned.

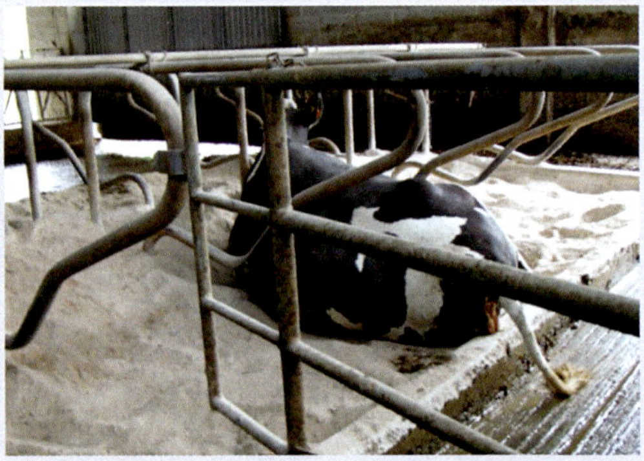

Figure 50. In many cases, part of a common area can be fenced off to prevent the movement of the animals, allowing better monitoring as compared with grazing dry cows.

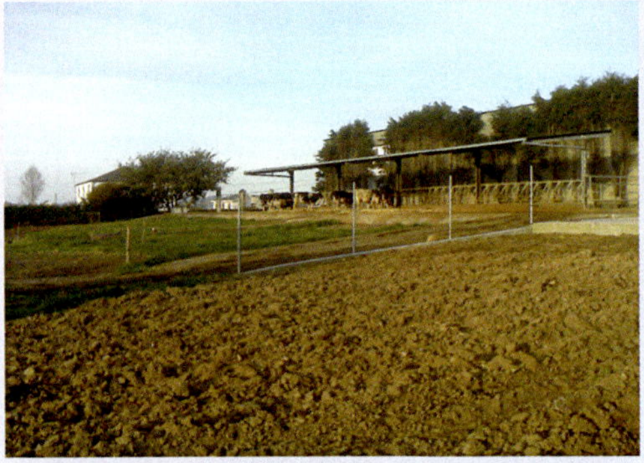

Figure 51. Dry cows can be kept at pasture as long as the grass is adequate and the animals are regularly monitored and provided with supplementary feed.

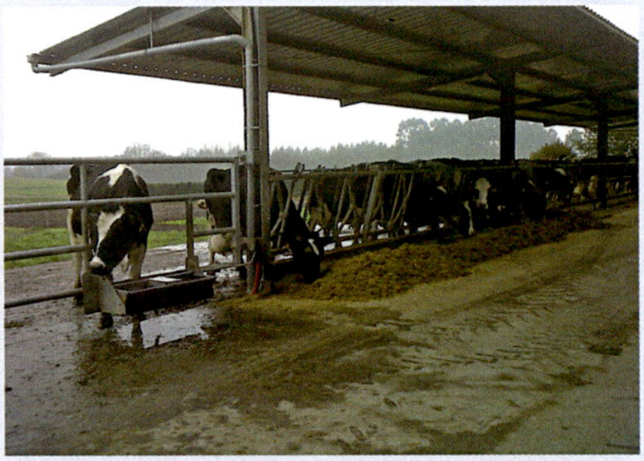

Figure 52. All batches of dry cows that are kept outdoors must be provided with sufficient feed and water of appropriate quality. Both feed and water should be protected from the weather.

to high-risk animals such as cows that become pregnant late or are diagnosed (by ultrasound) with twin pregnancies, cows with long dry periods and a high body condition score, and those that produce large quantities of milk and whose lactations are prolonged by the farmer, resulting in a very short dry period.

The following are some of the products and drugs that can be used to avoid postpartum problems: liver protectors, vitamins, glucose and calcium precursors, hepatic triglyceride mobilisers, essential amino acids (which promote liver metabolism). It is also recommended to monitor postpartum animals daily. All measures and protocols implemented by the farmer must be first reviewed by an experienced veterinary surgeon (Fig. 54).

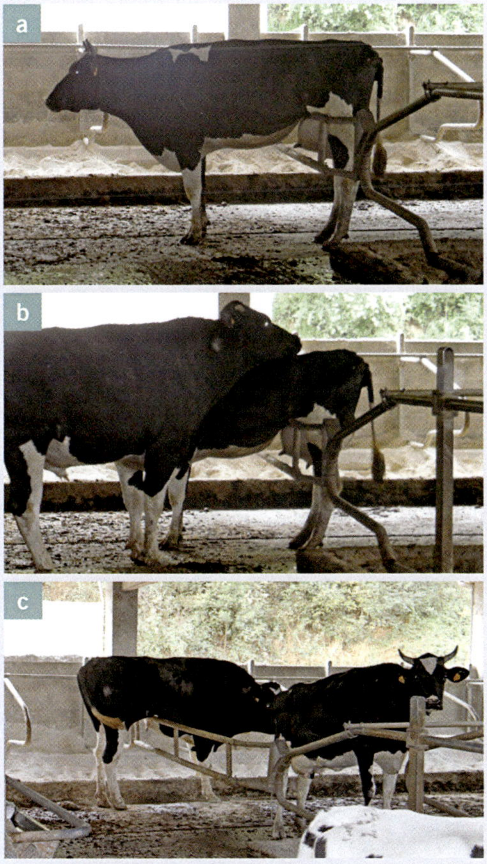

Figure 53. It is important to correctly separate batches of animals. For example, a bull should never be taken near the dry cow batch, as instincts can literally transcend barriers.

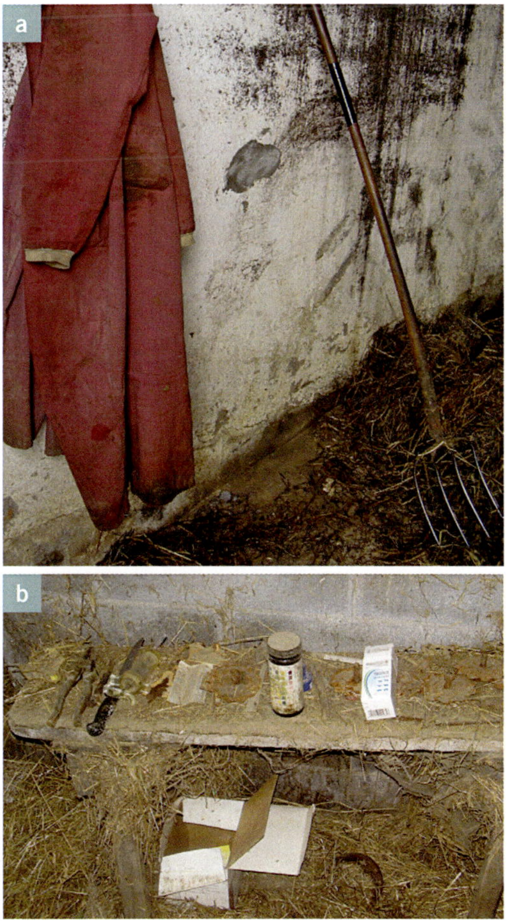

Figure 54. It is time to leave behind the image of the traditional, self-taught farmer and make way for a new, professional and well-informed livestock farmer.

7

Case studies

Case 1

Abscess in the hoof wall

Animal summary	
Age	4 years
No. of calvings	2
Production stage	5 days before estimated calving date

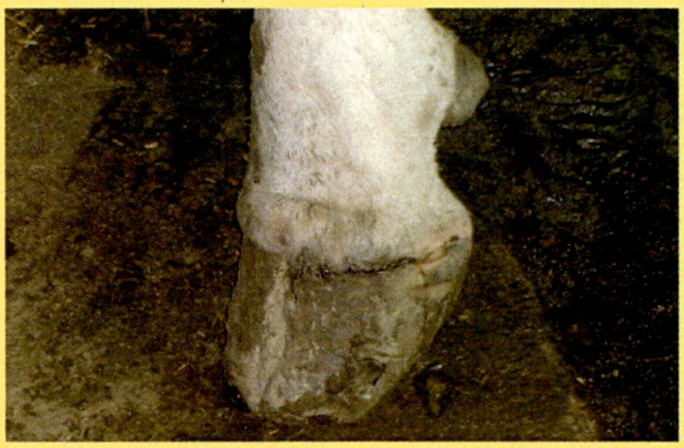

Reason for visit

The farmer notes lameness in a dry cow that is soon to calve. This female had been recently moved to the calving area for monitoring.

Anamnesis

The cow spends a lot of time lying on its right flank and presents acute lameness of the left hindlimb. In the preceding days no special attention was paid to this animal, even though it is soon to calve.

Examination and diagnosis

The animal has an abscess on the wall the hoof of the left hindlimb, the contents of which drain through the coronary band. The cow is diagnosed with severe lameness and left displaced abomasum (LDA).

Treatment

It is decided to induce labour and postpone surgical treatment until after calving. The cow is treated with:

- Intravenous corticosteroids: dexamethasone phosphate (30 mg).
- Natural prostaglandins (dinoprost, 50 mg), 12 hours after corticosteroid administration.
- Preventative antibiotic (amoxicillin trihydrate, 750 mg/48 h in 3 doses) for potential placental retention and given the likely need for surgical treatment of LDA.

Progression and prognosis

Within 40 hours of starting treatment, the cow calves normally. As expected, placental retention occurs.

Examinations on the day of calving and the following day reveal that the previously diagnosed LDA persists. Forty-eight hours after calving, the LDA is surgically corrected and antibiotic therapy continued.

The following drugs are added to the aforementioned treatment regimen:

- NSAIDs for 4 days: ketoprofen, 1.5 g/day.
- Natural prostaglandins (dinoprost, 25 mg) on postpartum days 4, 8, 12 and 22.

Twelve days after calving, the podiatrist is called to treat the hoof abscess. After performing curettage of the hoof wall (Figs. 1 and 2), the podiatrist attaches a hoof block to the interior claw of the left hindlimb, similar to that shown in Figures 3 and 4.

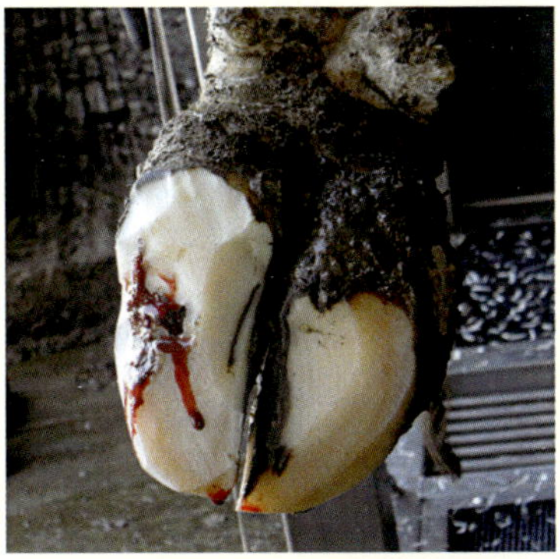

Figure 1. Ulcer located in the vicinity of the white line (normally, ulcers are situated more medially). If not treated, this injury will develop into a hoof wall abscess in about 15-20 days.

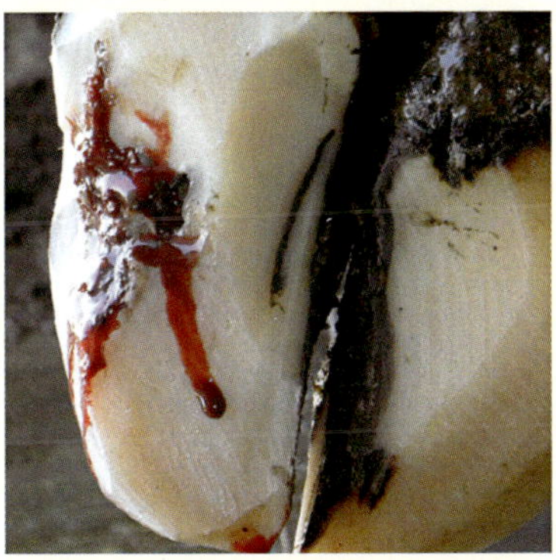

Figure 2. The logical progression of this lesion is the accumulation of fluid, which finds a route through which to drain, thus forming an abscess. Treatment consists of the attachment of a hoof block to provide better support to the healthy claw.

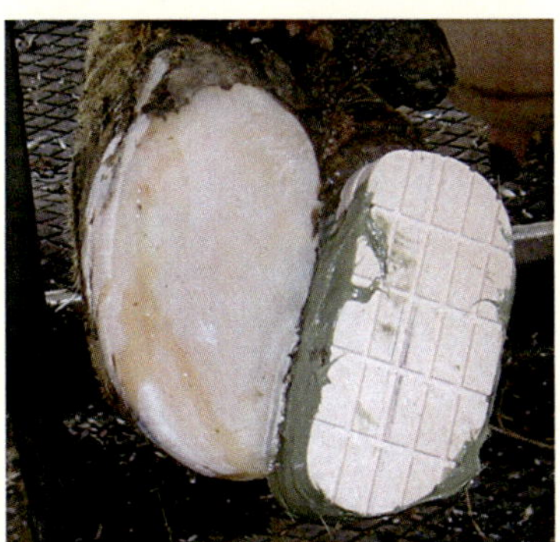

Figure 3. Injury similar to that described in the previous clinical case (Figs. 1 and 2). In this case, the injury is treated as soon as it appears. The hoof block has already been attached to the hoof claw. Fluid can be seen flowing from the vicinity of the hoof wall.

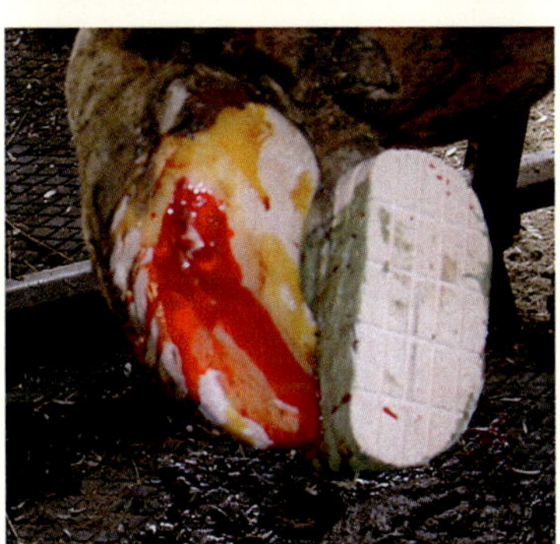

Figure 4. It was decided to open the hoof wall to facilitate fluid removal. Since the lesion was detected early, little damage has been caused.

REFLECTIONS

The data collected in the anamnesis show that the cow was lame at the start of the dry period, indicating that the cow was not properly monitored. At this stage of the disease, the diagnosis is an abscess of the hoof wall, which should be treated by a qualified podiatrist. With greater diligence, the initial injury could have been detected earlier and treated easily and inexpensively. However, in this case, the injury was left to develop into acute lameness with severe pain and the accumulation of pus, which drained from the coronary band. This situation was detected just before calving, which in turn triggered other metabolic problems (i.e. LDA). This was an easily avoidable incident that triggered a much more serious problem for the animal. Drying-off is a short-term investment. In reality, it is the first stage of the next lactation, and failure to appropriately care for animals during the dry period can result in costly problems further down the line. It is particularly important to monitor lameness during the dry period, as treating lameness later rather than sooner can be much more costly. On the other hand, hoof treatments should not be administered to recently calved cows, given the instability of the hip caused by the physiological separation of the pubic symphysis during delivery.

Case 2

Lameness in a dry cow: the perils of inaction

Animal summary	
Age	3 years
No. of calvings	2
Production stage	Pregnant (7.5 months) and reaching the end of the dry period

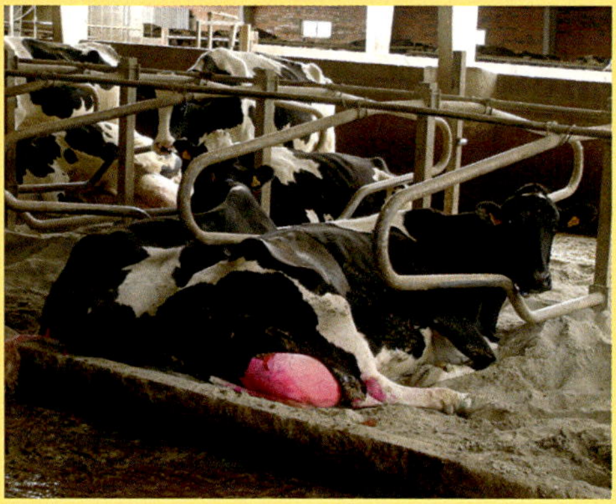

Reason for visit

On a routine visit to the dry cow yard of a farm, the vet observes a cow with a very noticeable limp.

Anamnesis

The state of the cow and its body condition score are appropriate for its production stage (dry period). The animal is limping noticeably and spends a lot of time lying down. On detecting the problem, a foot examination is recommended to the owner to diagnose the specific disease, but the farmer refuses and insists on an alternative treatment. In line with the client's wishes, the cow is treated with antibiotics (ceftiofur sodium) and NSAIDs.

The farmer repeats this treatment himself four times before calving, in a misguided attempt to solve the problem.

Examination and diagnosis

After calving, the cow's body condition is poor, it is still visibly lame and it develops retained placenta and subsequent metritis. Furthermore, LDA is diagnosed two days after calving.

Treatment

LDA is corrected by surgery, post-surgical antibiotic therapy is administered, and the metritis is treated. It is necessary to wait 15 days to diagnose the foot problem and treat the cow in the cattle crush (Fig. 1). The cow is provided with fibre-rich feed and plenty of water.

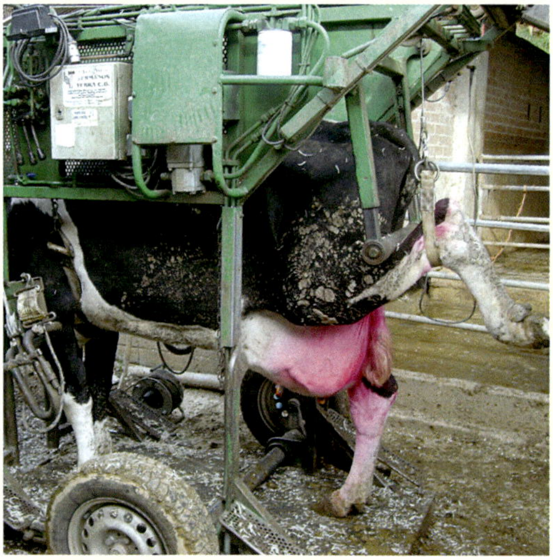

Figure 1. This disease should have been treated in the cattle crush once detected, when the cow was still dry.

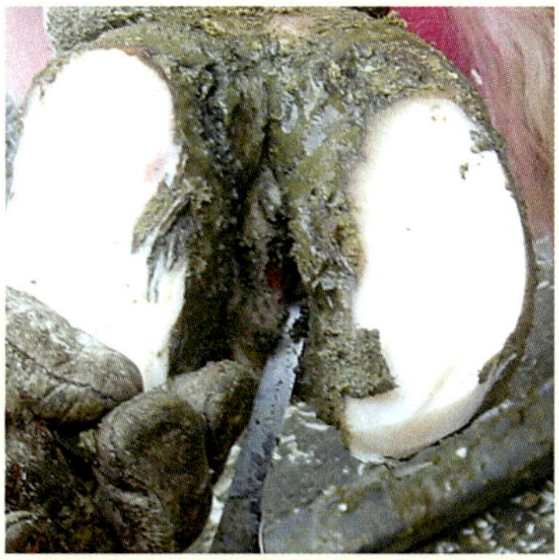

Figure 2.
A painful callus develops from untreated interdigital dermatitis.

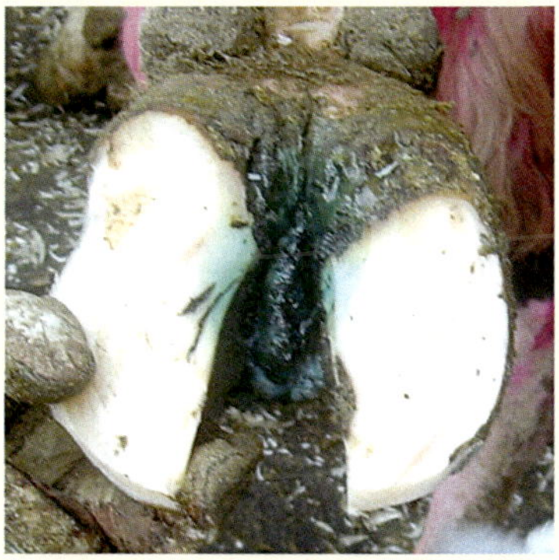

Figure 3.
In theory, this condition can be easily treated with cleaning, copper sulphate and bandaging.

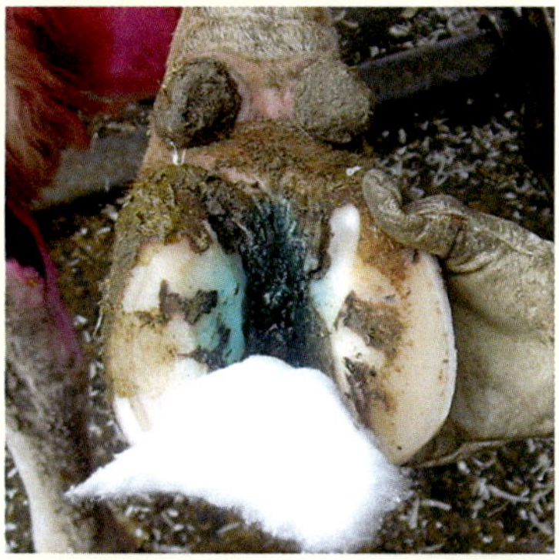

Figure 4.
As expected, the other hoof is also affected, although to a lesser degree.

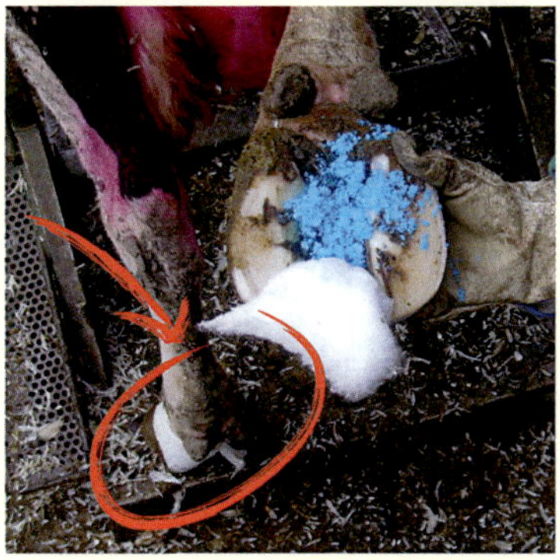

Figure 5.
The hoof problem is treated and a bandage applied to both hooves to ensure contact with the drug for 5-7 days.

Progression and prognosis

The animal progresses slowly after surgery due to multiple concurrent diseases (LDA, metritis, and lameness lasting 50 days).

Finally, the foot injury is treated (Figs. 2-5). After treating the callus that had formed, the cow progresses favourably, although the lactation peak is delayed and total production reduced.

REFLECTIONS

The lactation peak (litres produced) of this animal was much lower than expected, and thus the time taken to reach normal production was longer than the farm average. The medical treatment administered before calving was not ideal given the circumstances. Diagnosis and treatment of the foot problem was delayed, probably due to the farmer's apprehension about placing the cow in the crush.
All cases handled should be documented in writing by the veterinary professional for their records, always making note of the solution proposed initially.

Case 3

Left displaced abomasum complicated by surgical abscess

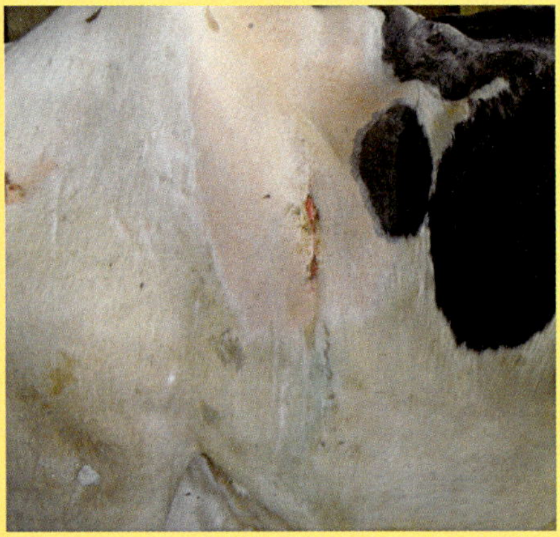

Animal summary	
Age	6 years
No. of calvings	4
Production stage	Postpartum day 4

Reason for visit

The farmer called the vet because a cow that had calved four days earlier stopped eating.

Anamnesis

The delivery was normal and the cow expelled the placenta, but milk production did not increase as expected. The female was milked three times a day and production recorded. The farmer thus noticed a slight decrease in production as compared with the previous day.

The cow's data sheet contains information on body temperature and treatment protocols administered by the farmer (Table 1).

Additional information

This cow belongs to an intensive farm, is housed in sand cubicles and has been milked three times a day since 2009. Feed is distributed by Unifeed cart. Females are closely monitored during the postpartum period, and relevant data recorded daily (Table 2). This farm has no prepartum batch. Note the length of the second lactation (461 days), which is followed by an interval of 523 days until the next calving (Table 2). The cow has a spectacular production in the second lactation and a dry period of the appropriate duration of 62 days. In April of that year (2009), the farm switched from two to three milkings.

Table 1. Postpartum data sheet.

POSTPARTUM DATA SHEET		
Cow identification no.: 2083 Day of calving: 20/03/2012		OBSERVATION Normal delivery placenta expelled
Days	Clinical data	Action taken
Postpartum day 1	Morning temp.: 37.8 °C	Intravenous Ca^{2}+ administration. Repeated 24 hours later.
	Afternoon temp.: 38 °C	Oral administration of propylene glycol and intravenous administration of vitamin complexes (daily).

Table 2. Production data sheet.

PRODUCTION DATA SHEET									
Cow identification no.: 2083									
Lactation Number	Birth date	TDR	Start of lactation	DM	End of lactation	Dry days	Actual production	CI	Litres/ day
1	09/08/2006	715	24/07/2008	306	25/05/2009	58	7,470		24
2			23/07/2009	461	27/10/2010	62	18,869	364	41
3			28/12/2010	329	22/11/2011	119	16,024	523	49
4			20/03/2012	1				448	
TOTAL		**715**		**1,097**		**239**	**43,353**		**39.5**

TDR = total days of rearing DM = days in milk CI = calving interval

The length of the next lactation, this cow's third, is normal (329 days) and the average number of litres of milk per day is very good (49 litres/day). However, the dry period following the third lactation is overly long (119 days). The cow stops producing milk earlier than desired. Coliform mastitis is detected at 104 days in milk, and becomes chronic, causing a sudden drop in production and earlier-than-expected drying-off, followed by a dry period of 119 days.

Examination and diagnosis

After examination, the animal is diagnosed with LDA.

Treatment

The LDA is corrected surgically, without further complications (Fig. 1). After surgery, the cow is treated with intravenous dextrose and vitamin B. NSAIDs are administered on the day of surgery and the following day. Antibiotics (penicillin and streptomycin) are also administered for four days.

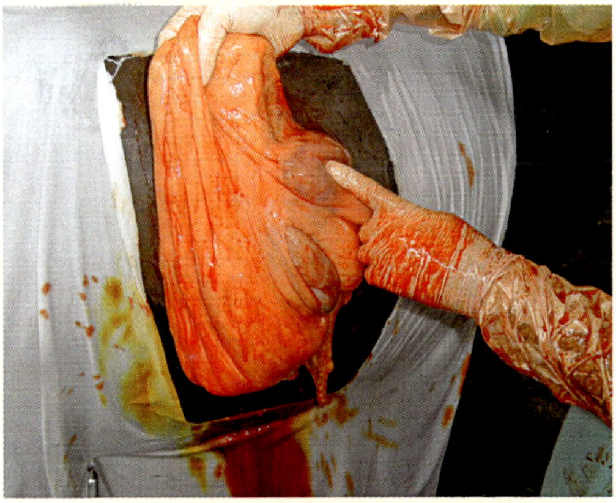

Figure 1. Externalisation of the pyloric sphincter.

Progression and prognosis

The cow is kept under observation for two days and is finally released after showing adequate recovery. Subsequent examinations detect no signs of ketonuria and normal temperature, production and feeding behaviour. In this case, all relevant animal and production data are recorded on the animal's data sheet.

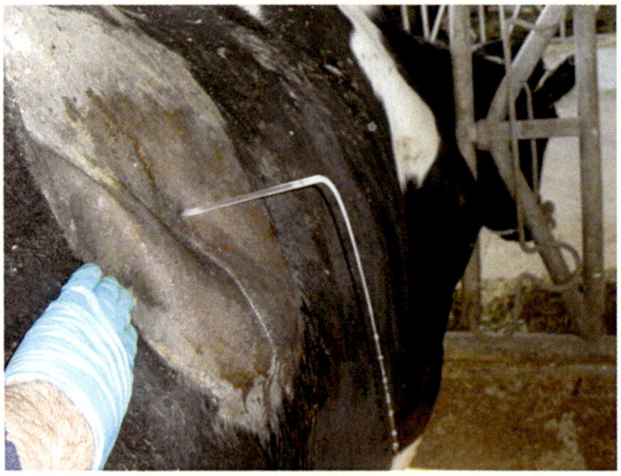

Figure 2. In case of a suspected abscess, an examination should first be performed, as described in this case report.

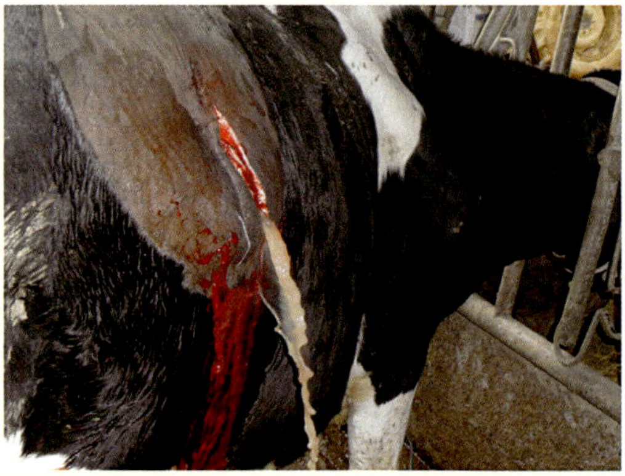

Figure 3. After surgical opening of the abscess, the contents are drained and debris removed by washing.

The progression of the cow is satisfactory, as also evidenced by the recorded data. However, 20 days after discharge the vet is called again because the cow's production has plateaued, and has even decreased slightly. Another examination reveals an abscess in the surgical wound (Fig. 2). The cow's temperature is 39.9 °C.

Before proceeding with the surgical treatment, the animal is sedated and the area surrounding the abscess disinfected. The abscess is lanced with a scalpel, drained and washed with warm, pre-boiled water and iodine. Finally, the wound is left open to drain (Fig. 3). NSAIDs are administered for three days. The farmer continues to treat the wound as described for a further seven days. As the abscess resolves, the cow improves and production increases.

Table 3 shows the changes in production and the diseases developed during the postpartum period.

REFLECTIONS

Postoperative complications are relatively common for several reasons: first, due to possible rejection by the organism of the suture material used, and second, due to a lack of hygiene/disinfection when performing surgery. Although many surgeries performed under sub-optimal conditions result in successful resolution, the clinician should not ignore these important considerations. In any case, early detection of any complications and swift and decisive clinical action is the best approach to successfully solving problems.

Table 3. Summary of the cow's production per postpartum day.

LDA (postpartum day 3)

Postpartum day	1			2			3			4			5		
Milking	AM	MD	PM	AM	MD	PM	AM	MD	PM	AM	MD	PM	AM	MD	PM
Litres of milk	9	6	8.6	9.2	8	8.2	8.6	6.6	7.2	8.8	5.2	7.6	9.2	6.8	8.2
TOTAL MILK		**23.6**			**25.4**			**22.4**			**21.6**			**24.2**	
Temperature (ºC)		37.8		37.8			38.3			38.2		39.2		38.5	

Postpartum day	6			7			8			9			10		
Milking	AM	MD	PM	AM	MD	PM	AM	MD	PM	AM	MD	PM	AM	MD	PM
Litres of milk	11	7.8	9	12	8.6	10	11.2	10.6	11.8	13.8	10.0	11.6	13.4	10.2	12.2
TOTAL MILK		**27.6**			**30.6**			**33.6**			**35.4**			**35.8**	
Temperature (ºC)	30.2	38.6		39.3			39.5			39.3			39.9		

Postpartum day	11			12			13			14			15		
Milking	AM	MD	PM	AM	MD	PM	AM	MD	PM	AM	MD	PM	AM	MD	PM
Litres of milk	14.6	10.4	12.0	14.8	9.6	12.6	14.8	10.2	12.6	15.0	12.0	12.0	14.8	11.2	12.8
TOTAL MILK		**37**			**37**			**37.6**			**39**			**38.8**	
Temperature (ºC)	39.4														

Postpartum day	16			17			18			19			20		
Milking	AM	MD	PM	AM	MD	PM	AM	MD	PM	AM	MD	PM	AM	MD	PM
Litres of milk	15.0	10.4	12.4	15.8	12.2	13.0	16.4	11.6	14.2	16.6	12.0	13.0	16.0	11.0	13.6
TOTAL MILK		**37.8**			**41**			**42.2**			**41.6**			**40.6**	
Temperature (ºC)															

Abscess treatment (postpartum day 21)

Postpartum day	21			22			23			24			25		
Milking	AM	MD	PM	AM	MD	PM	AM	MD	PM	AM	MD	PM	AM	MD	PM
Litres of milk	14.8	10.2	13.0	14.0	10.4	14.8	16.8	11.8	13.6	16.4	11.8	13.6	16.4	11.2	13.6
TOTAL MILK		**38**			**39.2**			**42.2**			**41.8**			**41.2**	
Temperature (ºC)		39.0		39.4	38.4		39.3			39.2				38.9	

Postpartum day	26			27			28			29			30		
Milking	AM	MD	PM	AM	MD	PM	AM	MD	PM	AM	MD	PM	AM	MD	PM
Litres of milk	17.0	10.2	13.2	17.6	12.2	15.2	17.0	12.8	16.0	17.8	14.2	15.2	19.8	13.2	14.6
TOTAL MILK		**40.4**			**45**			**45.8**			**47.2**			**47.6**	
Temperature (ºC)					38.7										

AM: morning MD: mid-day PM: afternoon

Case 4

Drying-off and social relationships

Animal summary	
Age	5 years
No. of calvings	3
Production stage	Postpartum day 2

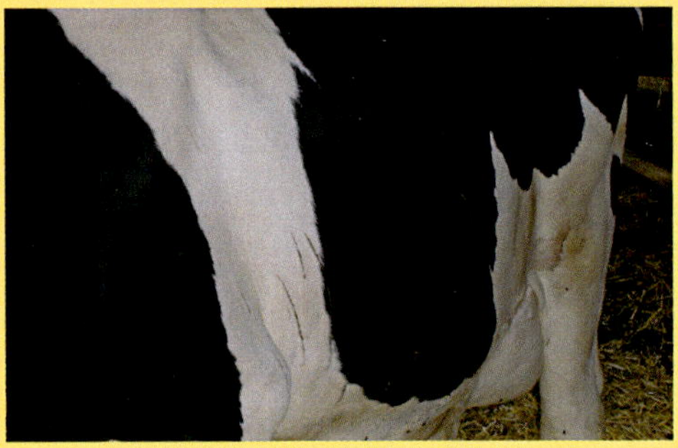

Reason for visit

The vet is called when the farmer reports a case of placental retention after calving. This cow had calved one week before the estimated calving date.

Anamnesis

The cow had calved before the scheduled date and presented retained placenta (Fig. 1). On performing the anamnesis, the vet notices that the drying-off area houses dry cows with heifers that have not been dehorned (Fig. 2). The farmer mentions that sometimes the heifers are aggressive towards the dry cows (Fig. 3).

Examination and diagnosis

Retained placenta is confirmed by visual examination of the cow. The cow's temperature is 39 °C. The urine analysis and all other parameters analysed are normal.

Treatment

Beginning on postpartum day 2, the cow is treated with antibiotics (ceftiofur sodium) every 24 hours for six days, and is injected with an NSAID every 24 hours for three days. Natural prostaglandins are administered on postpartum days 4, 8, 12 and 22.

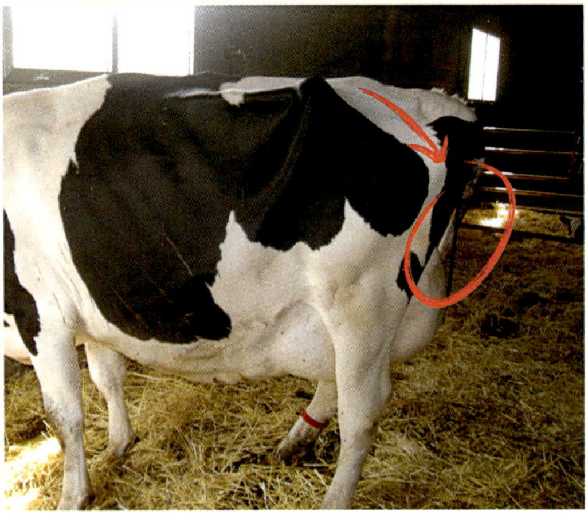

Figure 1. Note the horn marks in the rib area, and the exposed placental tissue.

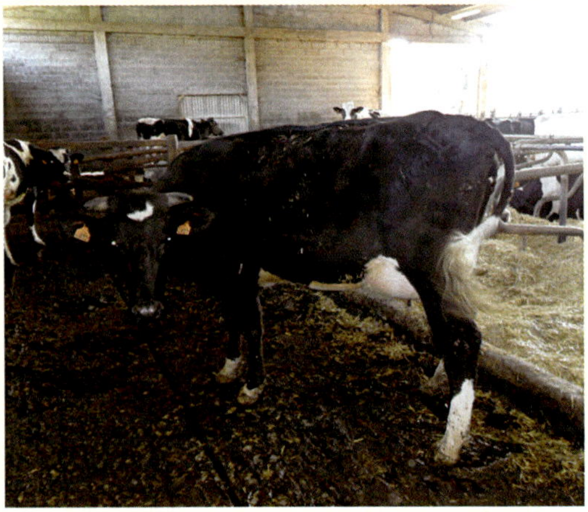

Figure 2. Animals should always be dehorned. It is especially dangerous to keep horned animals in the lactation area.

Progression and prognosis

The cow is monitored and reviewed every two days and progresses well. On the ninth day, the animal spontaneously expels the whole placenta. Another visit is scheduled to perform a uterine lavage, coinciding with the postpartum examination 20 days after calving.

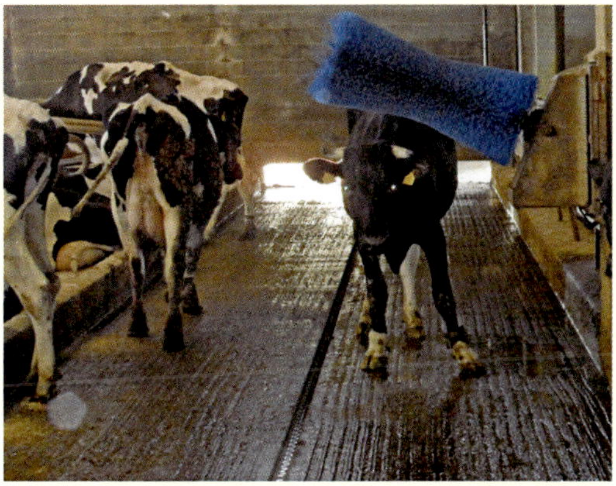

Figure 3. A horned heifer using the "anti-stress" brush.

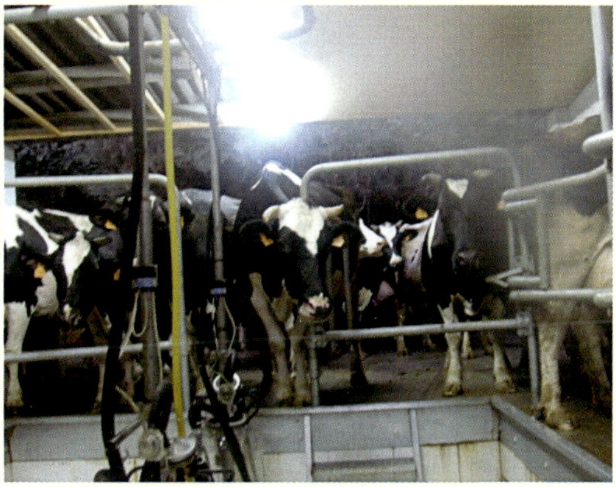

Figure 4. Horned cows in the waiting area.

REFLECTIONS

Exceeding the recommended age for dehorning (15-30 days) can cause problems later on, as illustrated in this case study. While this oversight may seem trivial, it is essential for the health and welfare of housed animals (Fig. 4). The solution is simply to routinely dehorn animals at the appropriate age using the appropriate method (Figs. 5-7).

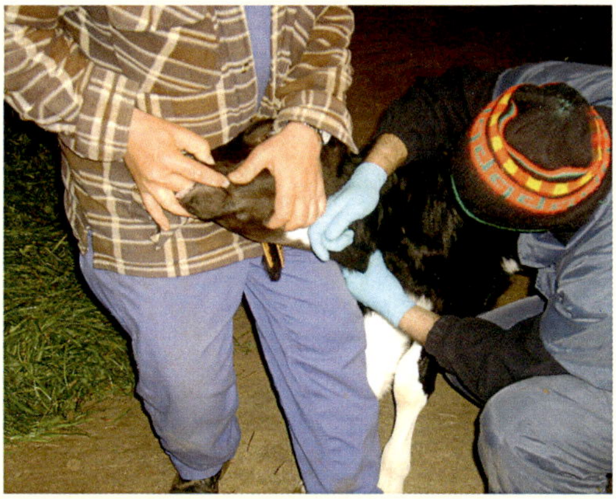

Figure 5. When dehorning, regardless of the method used, cows should first be sedated.

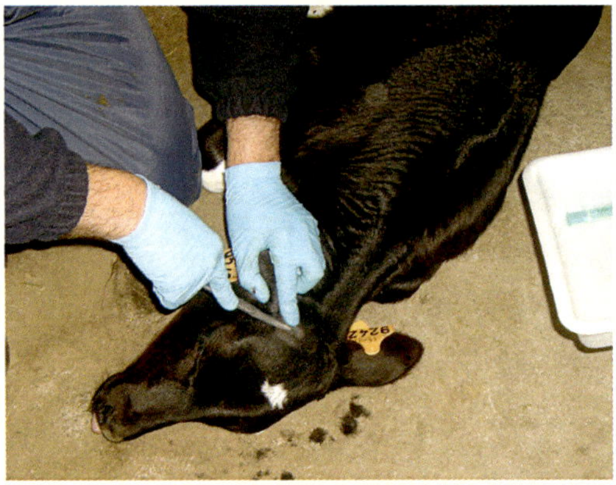

Figure 6. The optimal time for dehorning is in the first 15-30 days of life of the calf, as the procedure is easier and the animals more manageable.

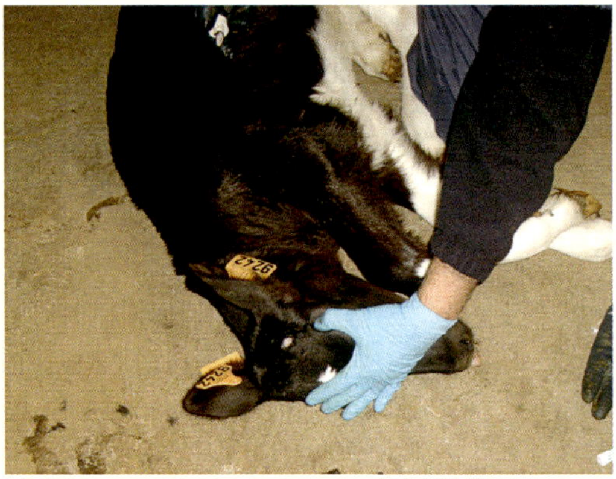

Figure 7. At early ages, the horn bud can be easily removed.

CASE 5 Perineal tears in first-calf cows

Case 5.1

Partial perineal tear

Animal summary	
Age	27 months
No. of calvings	1 (25.5 months)
Production stage	47 days in lactation

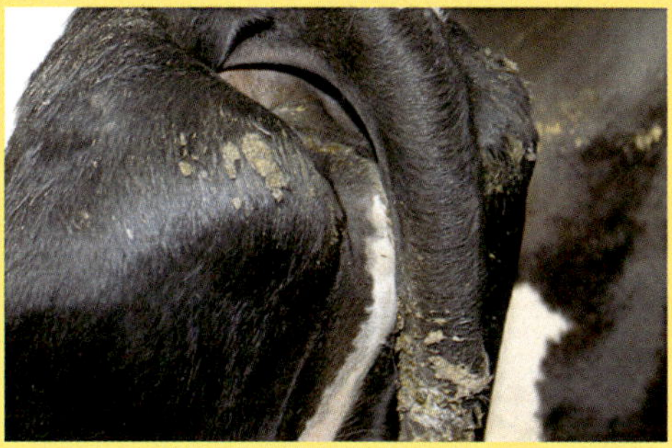

Reason for visit

On several occasions, the farmer observes white mucus on the bed on which the cow lies and notices that the cow holds the base of its tail aloft.

Anamnesis

The cow had calved in a delivery area with straw bedding and was lying down during the delivery. The assistants intervened in order to extract the calf's head, but otherwise the delivery was normal.

Examination and diagnosis

In this cow, the longitudinal axis of the vulvar lips is offset, and is practically horizontal (Fig. 1). Examination of the internal genital area reveals pneumovagina with an enlarged cavity and whitish mucus (Fig. 2). No tears in the vestibule are detected, although the internal wall of the perineum is weak.

This case is diagnosed on postpartum day 16. It is thus decided to wait until uterine involution is

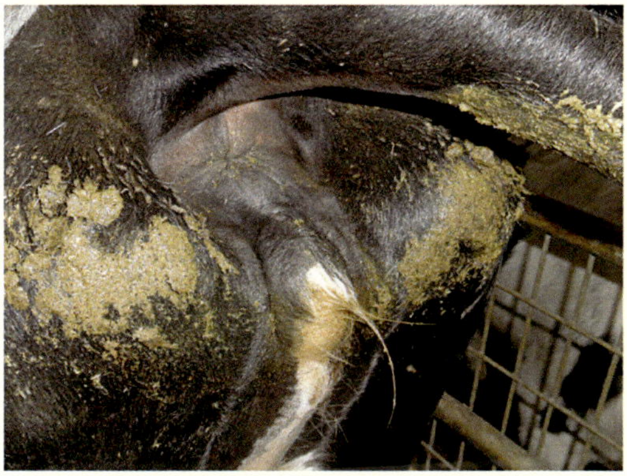

Figure 1. The longitudinal axis of the vulvar lips is more horizontal than vertical, which promotes pneumovagina.

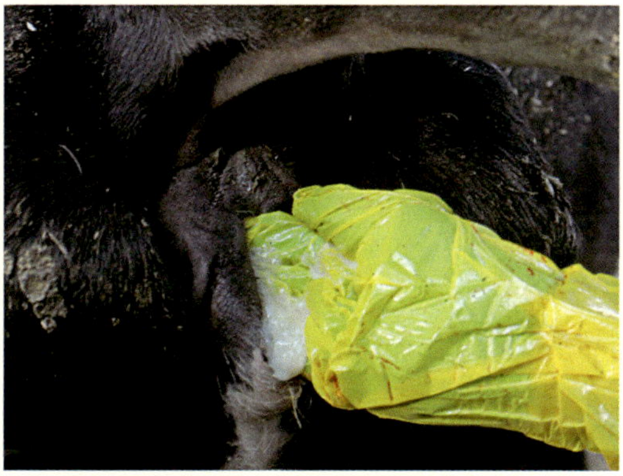

Figure 2. Examination reveals whitish mucus formed due to constant agitation of vaginal secretions due to the entry of air.

complete and to then reassess the situation. The initial diagnosis is subsequently confirmed and it is decided to opt for reconstructive surgery.

Treatment

A modified corrective pexis is performed to fix and strengthen the weakened tissue in the perineum. This technique involves obliquely cutting the top part of the vagina to bring the walls closer together and thus achieve a more vertical orientation of the area. The horizontal orientation of the vulva is such that a regular corrective pexis will not prevent the entry of air into the vagina (Figs. 3-12). Antibiotic treatment is not required.

Progression and prognosis

In general, the prognosis for this type of surgery is good (Fig. 13).

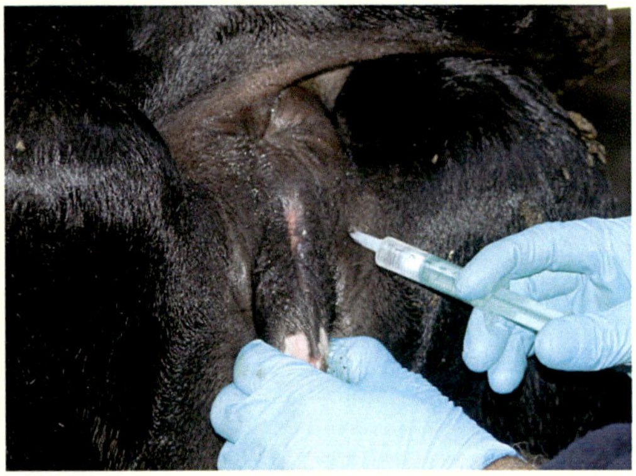

Figure 3. Epidural anaesthesia is administered followed by subcutaneous local anaesthesia.

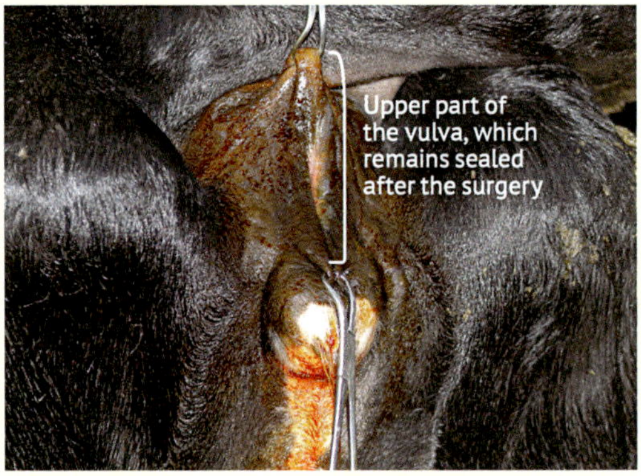

Figure 4. Prepared surgical field. The veterinary surgeon works on the upper half of the vulva to correct the pneumovagina while maintaining a normal opening to the vaginal cavity.

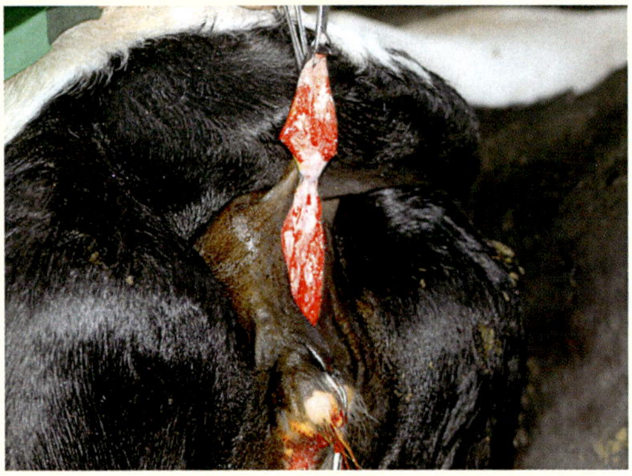

Figure 5. A portion of tissue is removed from the weakened area, cutting at an angle and dissecting deep tissue to strengthen the region with stitches. Joining the edges of the wound results in a stronger wall and a vertical orifice.

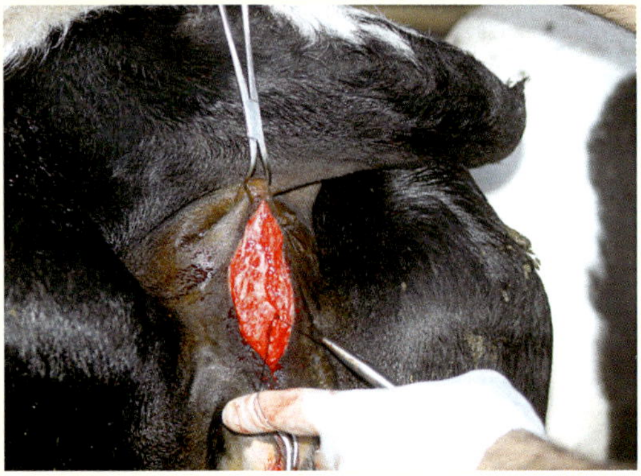

Figure 6. Beginning of the continuous suture. Synthetic polyglyconate 2-0 suture is used with a 40-mm long, ½-circle triangular needle.

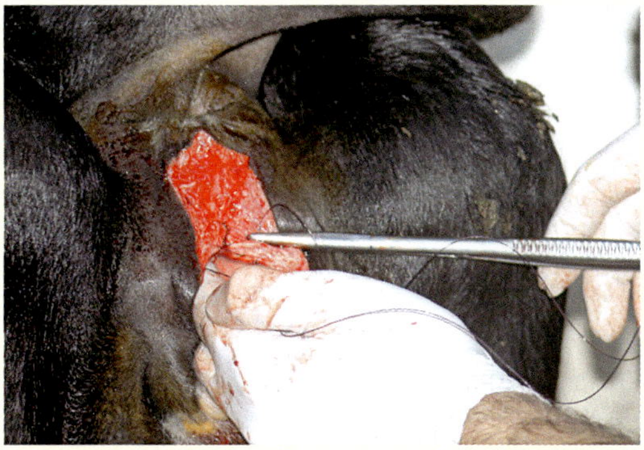

Figure 7. The first layer of the suture of the subcutaneous tissue runs from top to bottom in a far-near pattern until reaching the forceps, which delimit what will form the upper part of the vulva after surgery. As it descends, the suture forms a ridge that will be orientated towards the vaginal cavity. This suture closes the roof of the vagina. Care is taken not to pierce the vaginal mucosa.

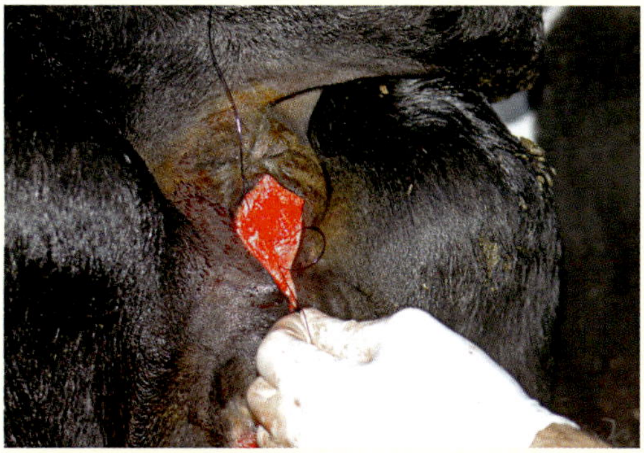

Figure 8. On reaching the bottom of the incision, the suture continues with closing sutures in the subcutaneous tissue from the bottom up.

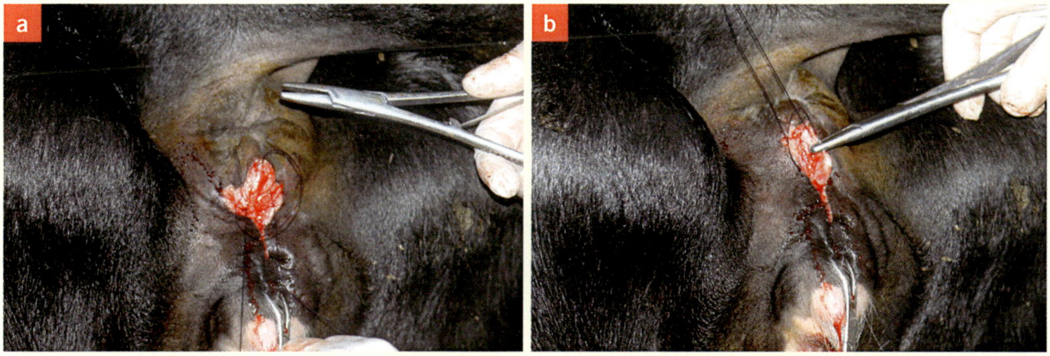

Figure 9. On reaching the upper edge of the incision, the suture descends again to strengthen the closure of the subcutaneous tissue.

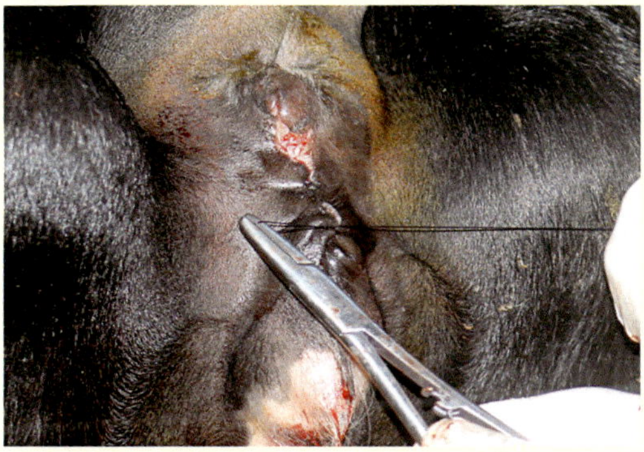

Figure 10. The suture continues from the bottom up, closing the cutaneous tissue with U-stitches. Finally, the suture thread is knotted.

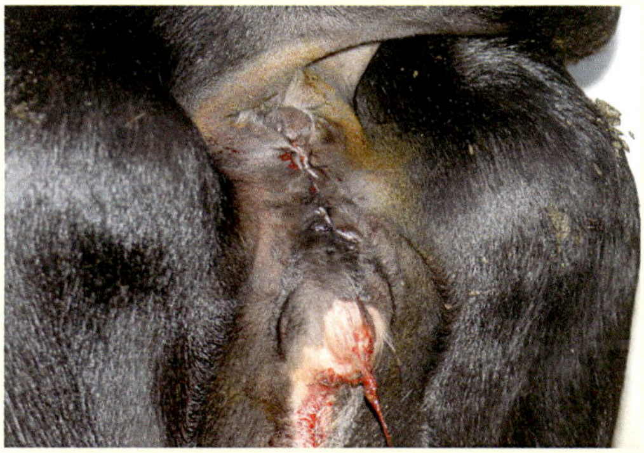

Figure 11. Two interrupted U-stitches are used to close the top of the wound.

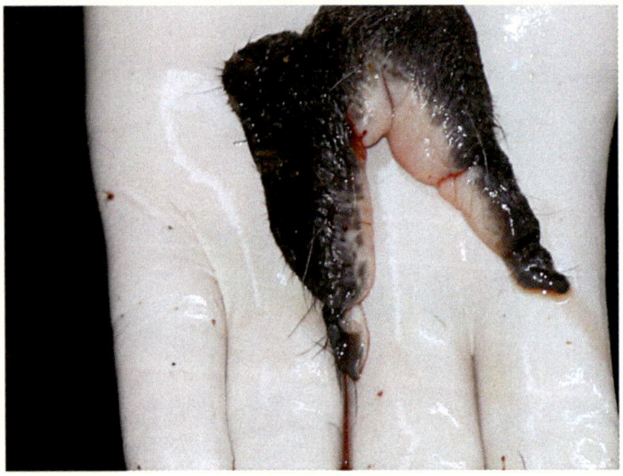

Figure 12. Flap of tissue removed to correct the defect.

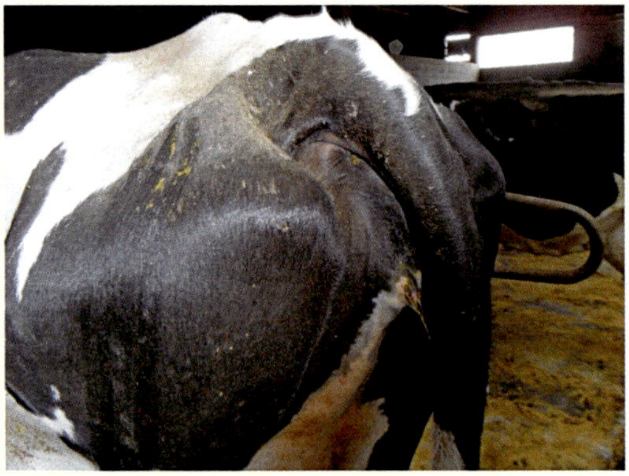

Figure 13. Revision 100 days after surgery, revealing good progress.

REFLECTIONS

Recently calved heifers often experience perineal tears, even after more or less normal deliveries. These conditions are due to physiological characteristics of first-calf cows, such as the width of the vaginal opening.

These cows are just beginning their productive life and represent the future of the farm. Moreover, they have not yet provided any economic return, and thus veterinary surgeons must be very careful during postpartum revisions when advising or taking corrective action. Neither the recently started lactation nor future gestation can afford to be compromised. As a rule, cows have not yet produced any economic return until they calve successfully and become pregnant for the second time.

To minimise the damage caused by these sometimes unavoidable conditions, it is recommended to closely monitor recently calved females, especially those that have calved for the first time. In these cases, early diagnosis and rapid resolution are crucial for the animal to develop properly, achieve a profitable lactation and become pregnant again, thus improving the overall productivity of the farm.

Case 5.2

Full perineal tear

Animal summary	
Age	25 months
No. of calvings	1
Production stage	25 days in lactation

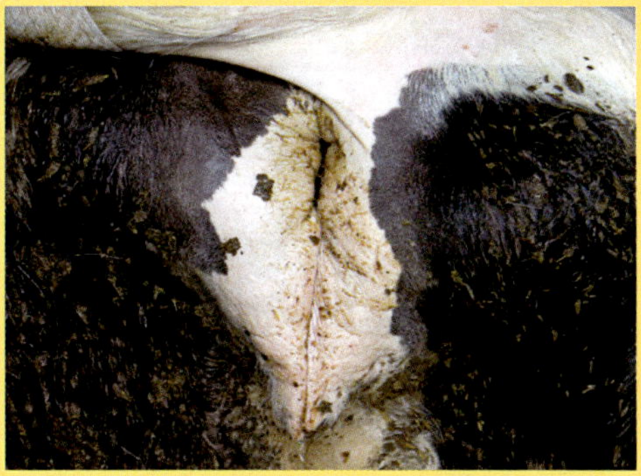

Reason for visit

The farmer is worried about a first-calf heifer that calved 25 days previously and is not eating. The cow is very irritated and straining continuously.

Anamnesis

After a near-normal delivery, the farmer, who intervened to extract the calf's head, notices a large tear in the perineum. The vet is called, and the wound sutured on the day of calving. The cow appeared to progress well for a few days, but the farmer notices that the tear begins to bother the animal again.

Examination and diagnosis

Examination reveals the absence of perineal tissue due to a complete tear that occurred during calving. The remains of the suture performed on the day of calving can be seen. The diagnosis is a complete perineal tear resulting in a cloaca (Fig. 14).

Treatment

As 25 days have passed since delivery and the cow is very irritated by the cloaca, it is decided to act without delay. Reconstructive surgery is performed to repair the torn perineum and resolve the cloaca. The objective of this surgery is to remove the old scar tissue and create a new partition of tissue that prevents the formation of the cloaca and forms a suitable perineum (Figs. 15-24).

The first step before beginning this intervention is to administer an epidural as well as local

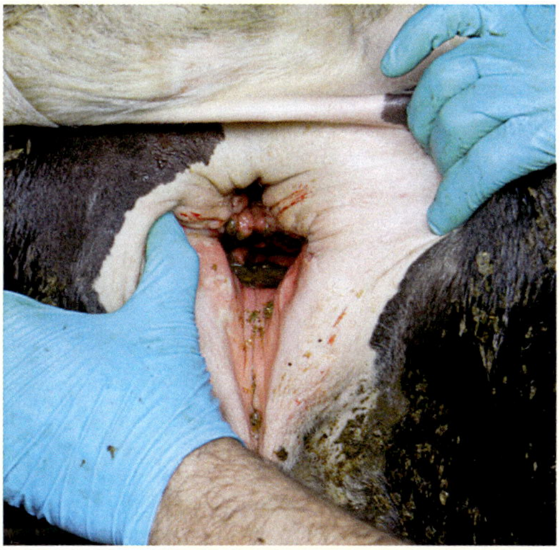

Figure 14. Separation of the labia reveals the depth of the tear and the resulting cloaca. Remnants of faeces can be seen in the vagina.

anaesthesia in the deep subcutaneous tissue (both vulvar lips and the region of the perineal tear). Before surgery, the area is cleaned and a towel wrapped in an insemination glove is inserted into the rectum to prevent the expulsion of faeces during surgery.

Using polyglyconate 2-0 thread and a triangular suture needle, a continuous U-suture is made in the rectal and vaginal mucosae. The stitches in the subcutaneous tissue of the new perineum are made using polyglyconate 2-0 suture thread and a triangular needle for the first interrupted

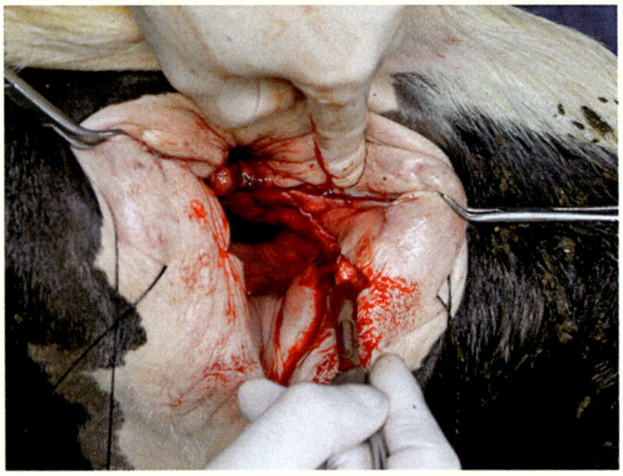

Figure 15. The incision is made in the deepest part of the tear, where the floor of the rectal mucosa and roof of the vaginal mucosa will be formed. The incision forms a triangle with its apex pointing inward, where the rectal and vaginal mucosae meet, and its base facing outward, where the new perineum will be created.

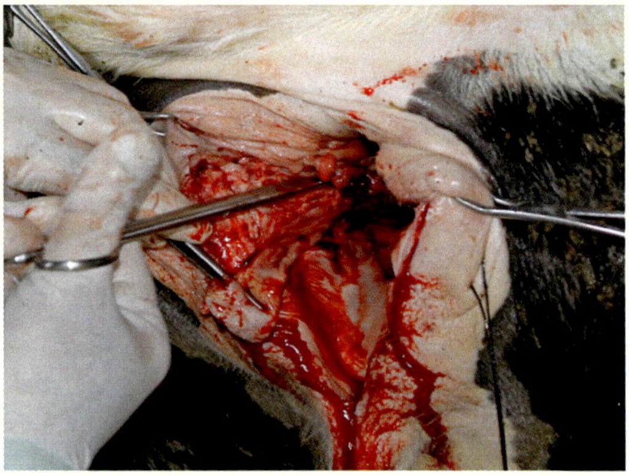

Figure 16. The scar tissue lying between the lines cut with the scalpel is dissected to reveal what will serve as the deeper layers of the new perineum. During surgery, the surgical field is frequently irrigated with saline.

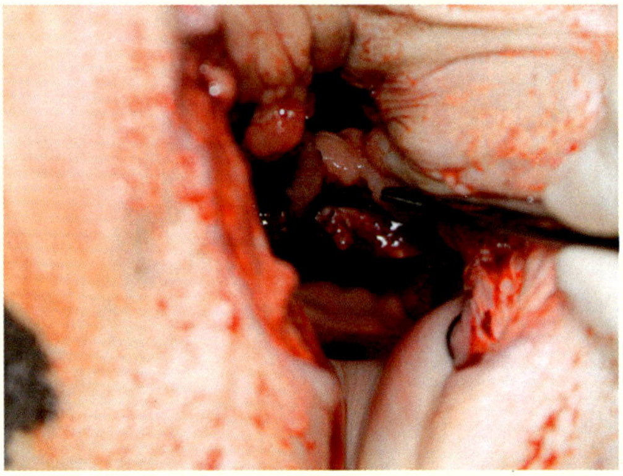

Figure 17. Note the apex of the triangular-shaped wound with the rectal mucosa above and the vaginal mucosa below. Between the two mucosae is subcutaneous tissue from which a separation between the two orifices will be reconstructed. This new partition is reconstructed from the deepest layers outward to the most superficial tissue layers (i.e. from the apex to the base of the triangle).

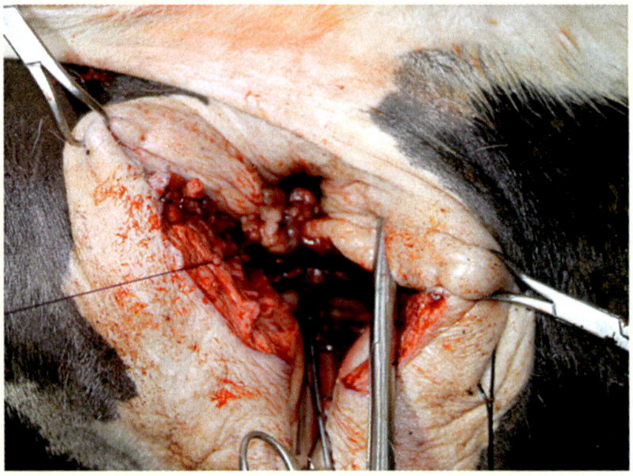

Figure 18. The vaginal suture begins (two stitches, conserving the remaining thread). Next, a continuous suture is made in the rectal mucosa (two stitches, conserving the remaining thread) and finally the suture proceeds to the intermediate tissue, from which the partition will be formed.

sutures. Chrome flexigut with an atraumatic needle are used for the most superficial plane of subcutaneous tissue, which is closed with interrupted sutures. It is important that the sutures fully close the incision (ensuring good coaptation with each suture) to create a solid perineum and to prevent the formation of fistulas. It is not necessary to administer antibiotics. In this case, the NSAID flunixin meglumine is administered for three days.

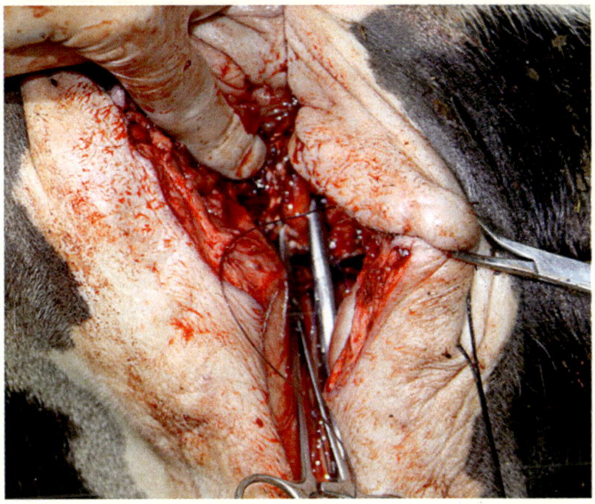

Figure 19. First interrupted stitches to draw the deep layer of perineal tissue between the two mucosae.

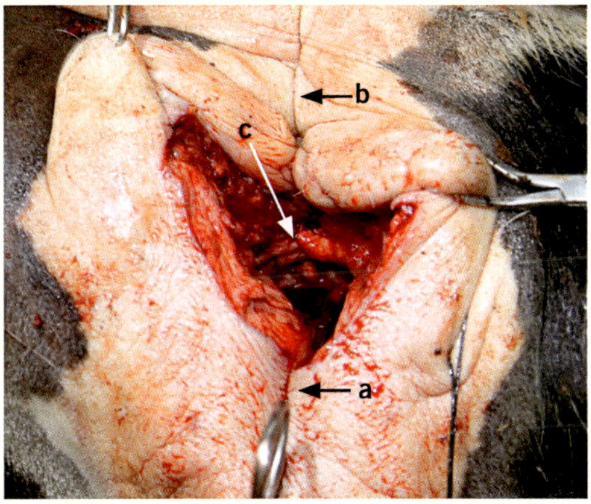

Figure 20. At this stage of the surgery, three different sutures can be observed: the continuous suture in the vaginal roof, the end of which is secured with mosquito forceps (a); the continuous suture in the rectal mucosa, the end of which is held by an assistant (b); and the suture consisting of the first interrupted stitches deep in the perineum (c).

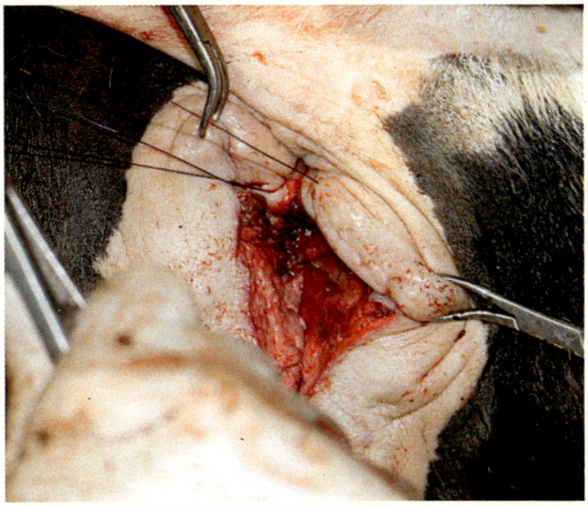

Figure 21. The suture continues with continuous U-stitches in the rectal mucosa. Note the closure of the subcutaneous tissue. The roof of the vagina will ultimately be sealed when joined with interrupted stitches to the tissue of the perineum.

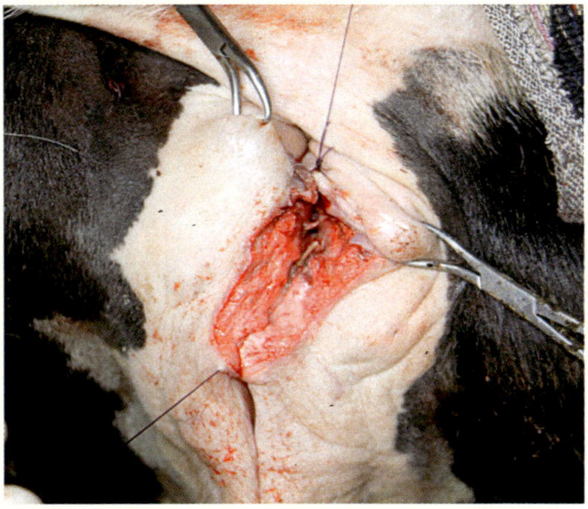

Figure 22. In the last step of the surgery, the sutures of the rectal and vaginal mucosae are completed, and tension is maintained while completing the suture in the perineal tissue.

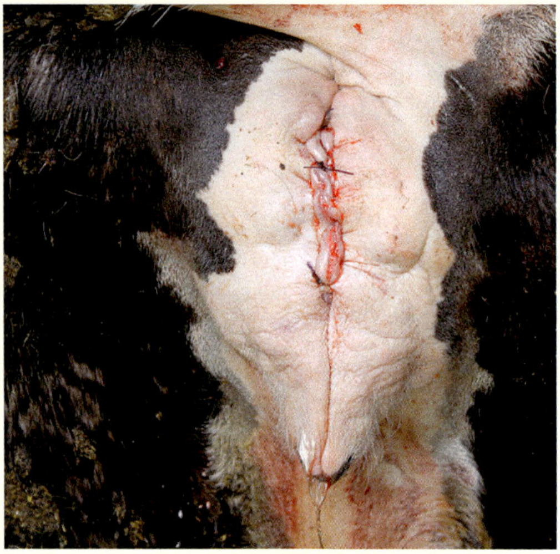

Figure 23. Result of the perineal reconstruction immediately after surgery.

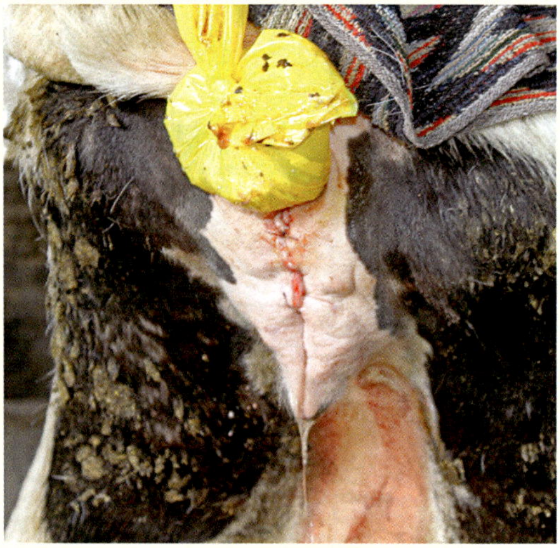

Figure 24. The glove that was introduced into the rectum at the start of surgery is removed. The new orifices created and the sealing of the rectal and vaginal mucosae are examined after surgery.

Progression and prognosis

After surgery, the cow improves markedly, stops straining, and is much more relaxed. The animal is examined 4, 11, 21 and 34 days after surgery (Figs. 25-28).

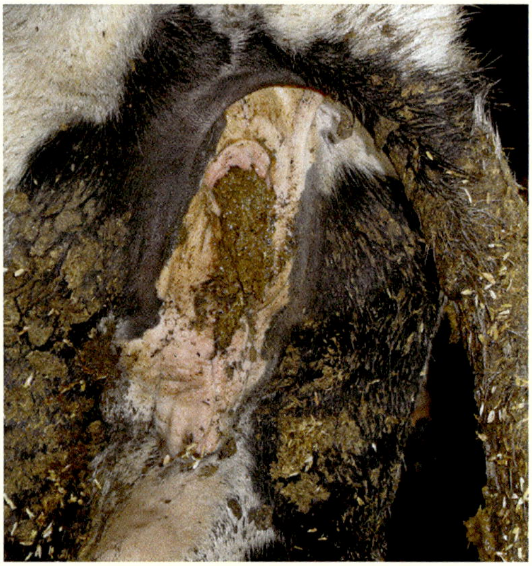

Figure 25. Revision on day 4 post-surgery. The vertical orientation of the new perineum is evident.

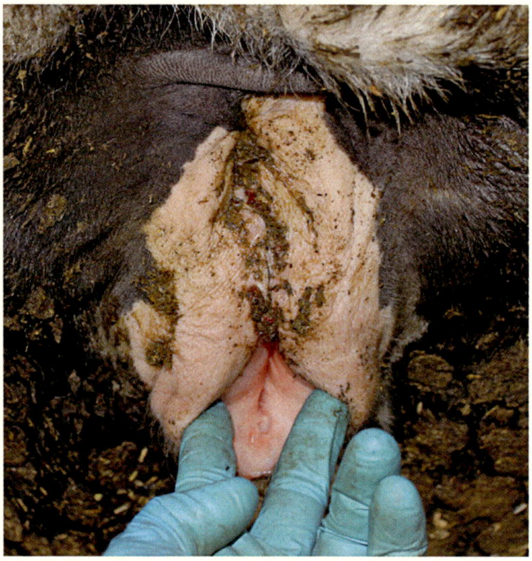

Figure 26. Revision on day 11 post-surgery. Progress is good with no inflammation of the tissues.

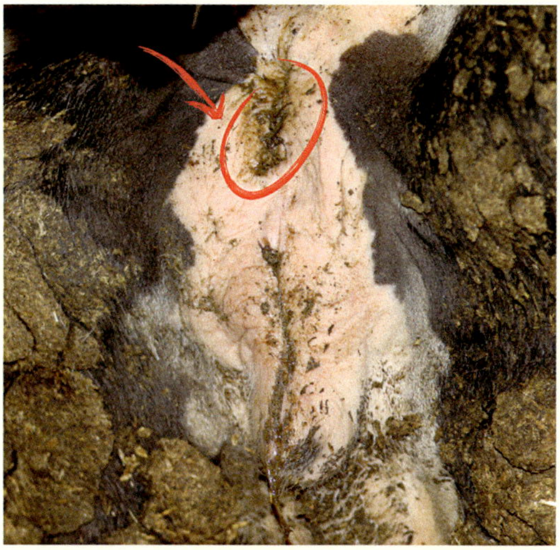

Figure 27. Revision on day 21 post-surgery. While remnants of the rectal suture can be seen, reabsorption of the perineal sutures has already begun (central cleft).

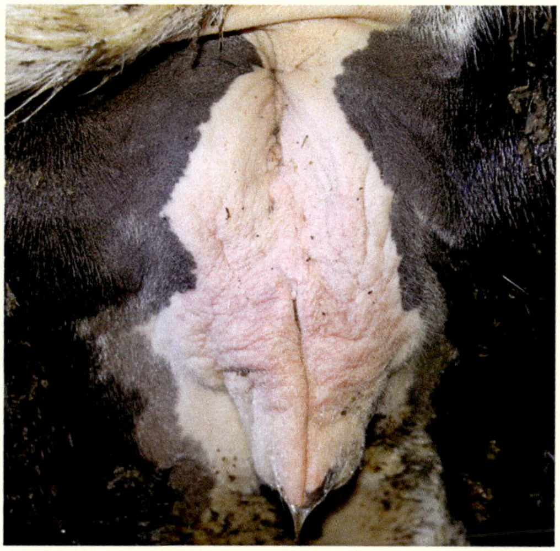

Figure 28. Revision on day 34 post-surgery. The vagina and rectum are examined once again. No fistulas are detected and the cow appears to have healed properly; the cow is released.

REFLECTIONS

First-calf heifers tend to have some degree of dystocia due to the narrow width of the vaginal vestibule, even when delivering small calves. In this case, the problem could have been avoided before delivery by performing an episiotomy, but the farmer did not anticipate a complicated delivery and did not contact the vet.

This surgery is less laborious if performed immediately after the problem arises, although the resultant oedema of the tissues can be inconvenient. In any case, we recommend acting early, always advising the farmer as to the pros and cons of the course of action advised.

Complete perineal tears are rare. However, when confronted with this condition, the professional must have at least a good theoretical grasp of the necessary surgical technique; this type of reconstructive surgery should not be attempted by the inexperienced.

Case 6

Multifactorial reproductive failure with complications due to anaplasmosis

Animal summary	
Age	7 years
No. of calvings	4
Production stage	Postpartum day 3

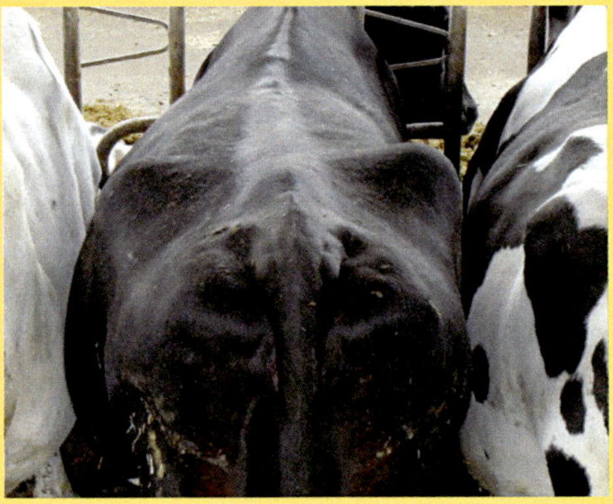

Reason for visit

The farmer calls the vet because a cow that had calved two days previously is apathetic, has a low temperature and hollow flanks. The cow has not improved even though the farmer has already administered the appropriate medication, following the relevant protocols.

Anamnesis

The anamnesis reveals that this cow, which has just calved for the fourth time, was dry for 100 days. Despite the cow's high production, the reproductive history reveals a very long calving interval (over 600 days), which explains why the cow has been dry for so long. The cow's body condition score during the dry period and around calving is higher than desired, but has not changed abruptly (BCS = 4).

It should be noted that the farm has a single production batch, and thus the ration received at the end of lactation is the same as that received in the earlier stages (Fig. 1).

The delivery was normal and the placenta was properly expelled. Following the farm's established protocol, the farmer had administered two doses (morning and evening) of calcium on the day of calving, and a dose of carbetocin immediately after delivery, both intravenously.

The following day, the farmer readministered the same dose of calcium along with 50 % glucose because the animal was cold and presented ketonuria (reactive strips were used to assess the presence of ketone bodies in the urine).

Examination and diagnosis

On the second day postpartum, when the veterinary surgeon examines the cow, it has a temperature of 38 °C, its skin is cold to the touch and its flanks hollow, and ruminal movements are reduced in intensity. The cow's milk production at the time is 26.6 litres. Analysis of ketone bodies in the blood reveals a score of 3.6 mmol/L of beta-hydroxybutyrate (BHB; normal blood BHB values should be < 1.2 mmol/L).

Based on the anamnesis and the treatment already administered by the farmer, the diagnosis is hypocalcaemia complicated by hepatic steatosis, which explains the high levels of ketosis and poor treatment response (Fig. 2).

Table 1. Data sheet showing relevant information on the productive and reproductive states of the cow in this case.

Birth	Artificial insemination				Calving			DM	Dry period		Production	Calving interval
	Date	Age (days)	Age (months)	AI no.	Gestation	Calving number	Date		Date	Duration		
09/12/2005	18/07/2007	1 586	20	4	2 216	1	19/02/2008	283	28/11/2008	55	6,795	
	18/04/2008	861	29	2	279	2	22/01/2009	494	31/05/2010	81	20,588	338
	16/11/2009	1,438	48	4 6	277	3	20/08/2010	536	07/02/2012	3 101	25,359	575
	09/08/2011	2,069	69	7	283	4	18/05/2012	301	5 15/03/2013		13,611	637
	29/01/2013	6 2,608	87	5								
TOTAL								**1,614**		**237**	**66,353**	**498 (Mean)**

TDL	2652
TDW	1614
TDR	802
TDD	237
TDU	1039

TDW/TDL	61 %
TDR/TDL	30 %
TDD/TDL	9 %
TDD/TDW	15 %

1. Becomes pregnant very late as a heifer.

2. Premature calving followed by lactation.

3. This abnormally long dry period can jeopardise the start of the next lactation.

4. The time taken to become pregnant for the third and fourth time is much longer than desired, and results in longer than normal dry periods (81-101 days).

5. This is the last entry on the data sheet. The cow has not yet been dried off. These data are used to calculate the DM (301) since the last delivery.

6. At the time of writing, the cow is pregnant. While not ideal, the cow's current situation is an improvement with respect to the previous calvings.

TDL: Total days of life
TDW: Total days worked
TDR: Total days of rearing

TDD: Total days dry
TDU: Total days unproductive (TDR + TDD)
DM: Days in milk

AI no.: Number of artificial insemination attempts required

Production/total days worked: 41.1 kg/day

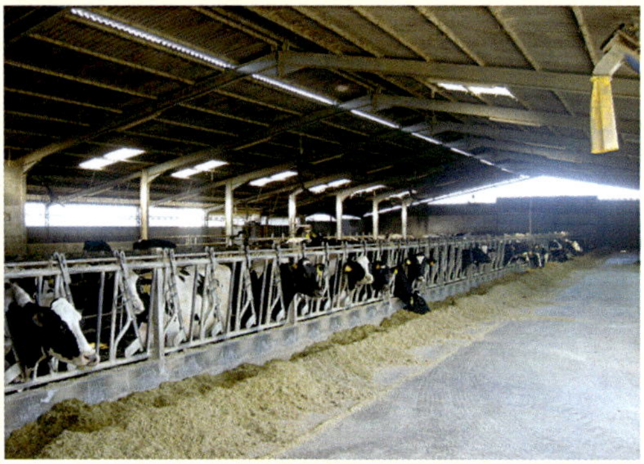

Figure 1. Most medium-sized farms on the Spanish Cantabrian coast have a single production batch, i.e. the same ration is administered regardless of the production stage of the cows.

Treatment

On the first visit (postpartum day 2), the veterinary surgeon begins treatment with calcium (administered intravenously that morning), as well as glucose, fructose and amino acids (acetylmethionine and arginine). Choleretic drugs (menbutone and phenoxy-2-methyl-2-propionic acid sodium salt) and B-group vitamin complexes are also administered.

In the afternoon, the vet examines the animal again and suspects a possible case of LDA. High levels of ketosis persist, in addition to the clinical signs observed in the morning. The vet administers a second dose of the aforementioned drug treatment.

The next day (postpartum day 3), the vet visits the farm, performs a complete examination of the cow and detects the following clinical signs: lethargy, body temperature of 37.6 °C, hollow flanks, absence of ruminal movements and few stools. Blood analysis reveals BHB levels of 3.1 mmol/L. The vet's suspicions are confirmed and LDA is diagnosed. Corrective surgery is performed without any complications. Furthermore, the cow is started on treatment with:

- Dextrose and amino acid solution, administered intravenously every 12 hours for at least 4 days. This regimen is maintained until BHB values fall below 1.6 mmol/L.
- Calcium diluted in saline every 12 hours on the day of surgery.
- Flunixin meglumine every 24 hours for 2 days.
- Choleretic drugs (phenoxy-2-methyl-2-propionic acid sodium salt) every 24 hours for 4 days.
- Propylene glycol (250 ml) every 12 hours for 1 week.
- Amino acids including carnitine, methionine and lysine, administered orally for 10 days.
- Antibiotic treatment (a combination of penicillin and streptomycin) for 4 days.

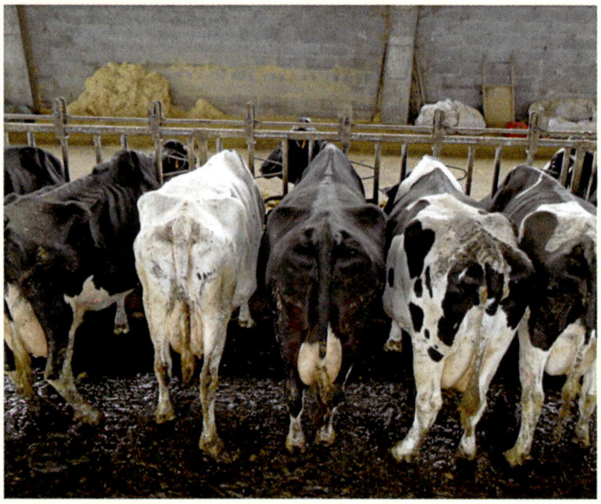

Figure 2. When a cow becomes pregnant later than expected, this creates a vicious cycle that can result in successive and/or concurrent postpartum diseases. This phenomenon is particularly prevalent on farms with a single production batch, where the difference between the actual energy requirements and feed intake is exaggerated. For this reason, cows with very different body condition scores can be seen in the same barn.

Clinical course

Table 2 shows the progress of the cow and the relevant production data. After surgical correction of the LDA, the milk yield improves, but stagnates again a few days later. BHB values are monitored (see Table 2).

At 16 days postpartum and after apparently recuperating, the cow exhibits a slight but progressive decline in milk production. On postpartum day 18, the farmer once again calls the vet, who examines the animal again, without identifying the specific cause of its condition. Rumination is maintained and while production decreases with respect to the previous days, it does not drop below 30 litres per day.

Production drops again on postpartum day 22. The vet detects tachycardia, mild fatigue, a body temperature of 39.3 °C and paleness of the mucosa, which is particularly noticeable in the vulva. The vet collects blood samples from the ear vein to perform a complete blood count to analyse the blood for parasites. Two days later, the test results confirm severe anaemia and the presence of *Anaplasma* spp.

At this point in the case study, we will briefly discuss anaplasmosis. Although rare in Northern Spain, the presence of this parasite is increasing in this region. In the present case, we suspect that the animal was incubating the disease for several days before clinical signs were evident.

From the day that the vet suspects an infectious process until blood test results confirm anaplasmosis, the vet prescribes the following treatment:

- Transfusion with four litres of blood, drawn from four healthy non-breeding cows that are in milk and have a BCS > 3.5. One litre of blood is drawn from each cow.
- Intravenous oxytetracycline hydrochloride (6 g/24 h for 10 days).
- Butafosfan.
- Vitamin B12.
- Iron every 48 hours for 8 days.
- Calcium diluted in saline every 24 hours for 4 days.

It is decided to omit one of the three milkings per day for nine consecutive days. The third milking is reinstated when production approaches 40 litres, to prevent the possible development of mastitis.

Prevention of anaplasmosis

Animals that develop and survive anaplasmosis remain asymptomatic carriers of the disease. Moreover, it is difficult to accurately diagnose these individuals without using specific methods. In our experience, a case of anaplasmosis on a farm in a non-endemic area usually indicates the start of an impending outbreak in other animals. Normally, anaplasmosis is transmitted by biological (ticks) and mechanical (flies, mosquitoes, horseflies) vectors, although iatrogenic transmission can also occur.

Young animals under one year of age that make contact for the first time with *Anaplasma* spp. are usually immunised, and exhibit few of the symptoms of the disease. Accordingly, the occurrence of infections should decrease over time as the percentage of immunised animals in the herd increases. In general, cases of anaplasmosis appear in the postpartum period, but they can occur at any time and even cause miscarriages in pregnant cows. To prevent the occurrence of anaplasmosis on farms, it is important to review the

Table 2. Summary of findings, actions taken, and production of the cow in this case.

Diagnosis and LDA surgery (day 3)

Postpartum day	0			1			2			3			4			5		
Milking	AM	MD	PM	AM	MD	PM	AM	MD	PM	AM	MD	PM	AM	MD	PM	AM	MD	PM
Litres of milk	0	0	8	0	6.4	9.2	11.4	7	8.2	9.6	6.6	7.4	7.5	4.8	7	8.8	7.4	9
TOTAL MILK		8			15.6			26.6			23.6			19.3			25.2	
BHB								3.6			3.1						3.6	

Postpartum day	6			7			8			9			10			11		
Milking	AM	MD	PM	AM	MD	PM	AM	MD	PM	AM	MD	PM	AM	MD	PM	AM	MD	PM
Litres of milk	9.6	9	9.4	10.4	9.4	10	11	8.8	10.4	13.8	9	11.2	12	11.2	10.4	15.8	9	13.8
TOTAL MILK		28			29.8			30.2			34			33.6			38.6	
BHB					1.8						0.6							

New decrease in production: maintain vigilance (day 16)

Postpartum day	12			13			14			15			16			17		
Milking	AM	MD	PM	AM	MD	PM	AM	MD	PM	AM	MD	PM	AM	MD	PM	AM	MD	PM
Litres of milk	14.2	11.6	13	14.4	10.6	13.8	16.2	10.4	12	14.6	11.8	11	12	10.2	10	12.2	11.4	10
TOTAL MILK		38.8			38.8			38.6			37.4			32.2			33.6	
BHB					0.6													

Postpartum day	18			19			20			21			22			23		
Milking	AM	MD	PM	AM	MD	PM	AM	MD	PM	AM	MD	PM	AM	MD	PM	AM	MD	PM
Litres of milk	11.8	9.2	9.4	11	8.6	10.6	12.8	8.8	9	10.4	8.4	11.4	10	6	8.8	10.8	7.6	8.6
TOTAL MILK		30.4			30.2			30.6			30.2			24.8			27	
BHB																		

management protocols. The following measures are recommended:

- Perform regular checks and establish rigorous prevention protocols against ticks that transmit *Anaplasma* spp., insects, flies and mosquitoes.

  The vectors that transmit this disease can be both biological and mechanical (Fig. 3).
- Use disposable needles and syringes on each animal.
- Do not share medication given to a sick animal with other animals.
- Bring dry cows indoors. This is the best way to prevent, or at least reduce, contact with the disease-transmitting vectors and other protozoal diseases (Fig. 4).

Much of the information available on this disease comes from tropical and subtropical countries, where the disease is endemic in cattle.

For this reason, many of the diagnostic strategies, prevalence studies, and treatment and vaccination protocols are not well suited to the characteristics the Iberian Peninsula (differential diagnosis with *Theileria* is particularly

Worsening of the process and clinical signs of anaemia: suspected anaplasmosis. Treatment and collection of samples (day 24)

Postpartum day	24			25			26			27			28			29		
Milking	AM	MD	PM	AM	MD	PM	AM	MD	PM	AM	MD	PM	AM	MD	PM	AM	MD	PM
Litres of milk	10	8.4	9.8	9.6	6.8	9.6	11	7.2	6.8	11.6	7.6	9.4	11	0	14.8	9.4	0	18.2
TOTAL MILK	**28.2**			**26**			**25**			**28.6**			**25.8**			**27.6**		
BHB	0.9																	

End of antibiotic treatment with terramycin (day 33)

Postpartum day	30			31			32			33			34			35		
Milking	AM	MD	PM	AM	MD	PM	AM	MD	PM	AM	MD	PM	AM	MD	PM	AM	MD	PM
Litres of milk	12.2	0	16.4	12	0	17.2	12.2	0	18	12.6	0	21.2	14.2	0	21.2	14.6	0	21
TOTAL MILK	**28.6**			**29.2**			**30.2**			**33.8**			**35.4**			**35.6**		
BHB																		

Postpartum day	36			37			38			39		
Milking	AM	MD	PM	AM	MD	PM	AM	MD	PM	AM	MD	PM
Litres of milk	16	0	16	16	10.8	12.6	16.6	9.8	13	15	9.3	14.4
TOTAL MILK	**32**			**39.4**			**39.4**			**38.7**		
BHB												

AM: morning MD: mid-day PM: afternoon

important as they are difficult to distinguish clinically).

In conclusion, a fast and reliable diagnostic method is needed. Moreover, a thorough study of the prevalence of these diseases should be performed to promote training and increase knowledge of emerging diseases, focusing on disease evolution and the factors that influence disease development.

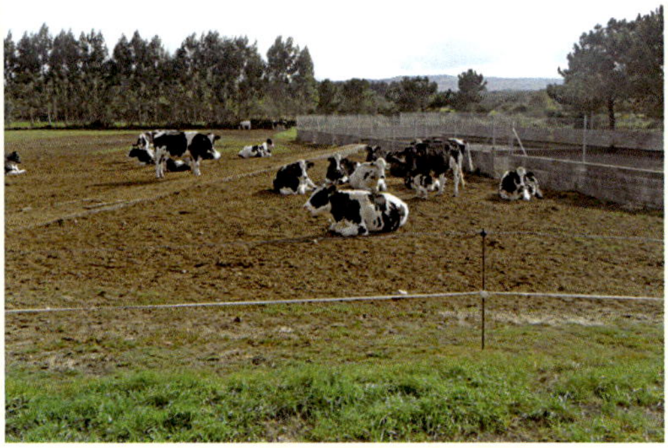

Figure 3. Outdoor areas can be pleasant for the cows, but are also dangerous due to increased exposure to ticks or other vectors of diseases.

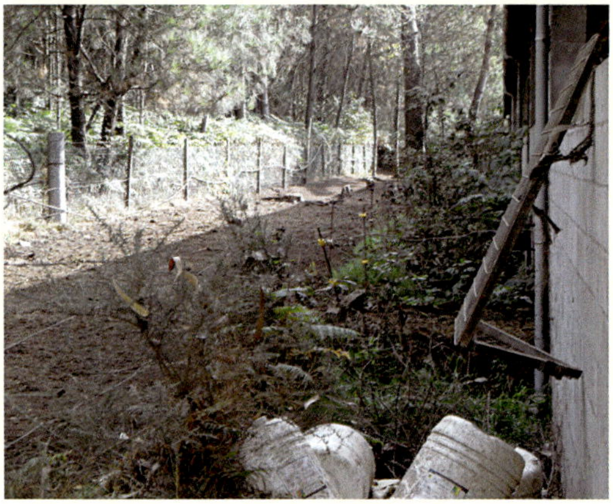

Figure 4. The outer wall of this farm has abundant adjacent vegetation, which can act as a reservoir for ticks that transmit anaplasmosis.

REFLECTIONS

This case is a good example of how a reproductive failure influences the length of the dry period and the body condition of the cow, which in turn can lead to subsequent disease that delay the next pregnancy. This domino effect thus creates a vicious circle that increases the chances of reproductive failure. Consider the following questions: should this cow not have been impregnated at that point in time?; is it necessary to strictly adhere to the deadline (days in milk) for insemination? In the present case, it is possible that the exceptional production of the cow justifies the farmer's decision, but in general such cases are uncommon. There are certain recommended guidelines indicating the time point up to which cows can be inseminated, depending on the production, days in milk, and the calving number of the cow in question.

In general, the work of the vet on the farm should be standardised as much as possible, using pre-established protocols and treatments. Often however, specific cases do not correspond to the guidelines; this is when the veterinary surgeon must act quickly, employing either surgical or pharmacological treatments, or checking for errors in the protocol in question. Can vets specialise while at the same time providing rapid solutions? Is there such a thing as multidisciplinary work?

Regarding anaplasmosis, remember that vector-borne diseases, whether biological or mechanical, are increasingly diagnosed in temperate areas although many of these diseases were previously considered tropical (e.g. bluetongue). The reasons for these variations are not entirely fully understood, but may include climate change and the adaptation of new vectors. What changes lie ahead in terms of the way veterinary surgeons are trained?

Case 7

Outbreak of acute clinical mastitis on a farm

Farm summary	
Type of production	Dairy
No. of cows milked	54
Comments	To reach a diagnosis, it is necessary to evaluate the entire production process

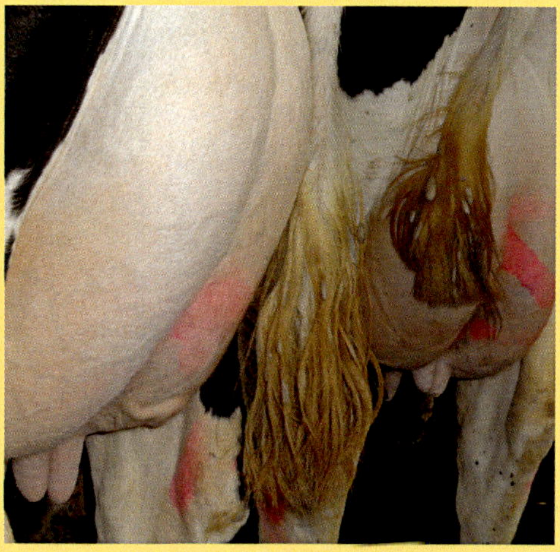

Reason for visit

The farm owner calls the vet after detecting an acute outbreak of clinical mastitis in the month of July.

Anamnesis

Eight cases of acute clinical mastitis are detected on the farm in July; two of these are fatal, and the other six animals exhibit a marked decrease in production.

The disease affects cows of all ages and all stages of lactation. Mastitis is characterised by inflammatory processes affecting one or several quarters, with symptoms of systemic infection that can have serious health consequences for affected cows. In animals that survive mastitis, the udder atrophies and pre-mastitis production levels are not restored. Milk quality is also significantly affected in cows with mastitis. Overall, a decrease in the production of the herd is observed, which is attributed to mastitis and an incorrect mix of concentrate given to the cows 15 days beforehand. The ration is distributed from a Unifeed cart, and was rejected by the animals on two consecutive days. This batch of feed was returned to the supplier.

This farm keeps a record of reproductive data, which provides an overview of the seasonality of calving. Thirteen cows calved in the month of July. These records also reveal a high incidence of postpartum disorders, including placental retention, hypocalcaemia and metritis.

The farm has established a good drying-off protocol, including preventative intramammary antibiotic therapy, antiparasitic treatment, and vaccination.

Tables 1 and 2 show data relating to the udder health of the animals and other data recorded during milk inspections performed on the farm. These data reveal:

- A high prevalence of animals with cell counts > 200,000 cells/ml.
- An increased likelihood of infection, i.e. there has been an increase in the number of cows that had cell counts < 200,000 cells/ml in one inspection and > 200,000 cells/ml in the subsequent inspection.

Table 1. Udder health and milking inspection data.

RECENT DATA

Date of last inspection	No. of cows on farm	No. of calvings	No. of cows analysed	1 No. of cows affected since last inspection	No. of cows cured since last inspection	2 Cows with chronic mastitis
25/07/12	54	47	42	3	4	4 (7.41 %)

HISTORY

Linear Score (LS)	Mean production	Percentage of animals > 200,000 cells/ml	Percentage animals > 1,000,000 cells/ml in last inspection	LS of heifers in first inspection	3 Percentage of heifers affected in first inspection	Percentage healed during dry period	Percentage of new infections during dry period
2.26	32.2	20.37 %	3.70 %	1.59	31.25 %	50 %	37.50 %
< 3		< 20 %	< 5 %	< 2	< 12 %	> 75 %	< 10 %

Date of inspection	No. of animals	No. of heifers	No. cows	Percentage of heifers	Percentage of cows	Heifer/cow ratio	Percentage of heifers > 200,000 cells/ml	No. of calvings
28/11/11	55	18	37	32.73 %	67.27 %	4.9/10	11.11 %	2
28/12/11	50	19	31	38 %	62 %	6.1/10	5.26 %	3
25/01/12	52	19	33	36.54 %	63.46 %	5.8/10	10.53 %	6
27/02/12	56	20	36	35.71 %	64.29 %	5.6/10	10 %	8
27/03/12	57	21	36	36.84 %	63.16 %	5.8/10	14.29 %	4
26/04/12	54	21	33	38.89 %	61.11 %	6.4/10	0 %	6
25/05/12	50	20	30	40 %	60 %	6.7/10	10 %	2
25/06/12	48	19	29	39.58 %	60.42 %	6.6/10	10.53 %	3
25/07/12	54	21	33	38.89 %	61.11 %	6.4/10	9.52 %	13
			Mean	37.46 %	62.54 %	6.0/10	9.03 %	4 47

Date of inspection	No. of animals	No. of animals > 200,000 cells/ml	No. of heifers > 200,000 cells/ml	No. of cows > 200,000 cells/ml	No. of cows > 1,000,000 cells/ml	Percentage animals > 200,000 cells/ml	Percentage animals > 1,000,000 cells/ml
28/11/11	55	14	2	12	4	25.45 %	7.27 %
28/12/11	50	10	1	9	1	20 %	2 %
25/01/12	52	15	2	13	3	28.85 %	5.77 %
27/02/12	56	11	2	9	1	19.64 %	1.79 %
27/03/12	57	14	3	11	3	24.56 %	5.26 %
26/04/12	54	8	0	8	1	14.81 %	1.85 %
25/05/12	50	8	2	6	2	16.00 %	4 %
25/06/12	48	10	2	8	2	20.83 %	4.17 %
25/07/12	54	11	2	9	2	20.37 %	3.70 %
					Mean	21.17 %	3.98 %

Mean days in milk at drying-off, based on the last inspection before calving	306
Correction factor	30
Total	336

1 Increased likelihood of mastitis infection.
2 Increased rate of chronic mastitis.
3 High percentage of heifers with mastitis at calving.
4 Seasonality of calving.

Table 2. Information on the number of cows with mastitis between 0 and 30 days in milk (DM).

Date of inspection	No. of cows being milked	Cows at 0-30 DM	Affected cows > 200,000 cells/m	Percentage of cows at 0-30 DM	Percentage of affected cows at 0-30 DM
28/11/11	55	6	1	10.91 %	16.67 %
28/12/11	50	5	2	10 %	40 %
25/01/12	52	9	4	17.31 %	44.44 %
27/02/12	56	14	5	25 %	35.71 %
27/03/12	57	12	4	21.05 %	33.33 %
26/04/12	54	8	0	14.81 %	0 %
25/05/12	50	6	3	12 %	50 %
25/06/12	48	4	2	8.33 %	50 %
25/07/12	54	15	5	27.78 %	1 33.33 %

1 High percentage of infected cows at 0-30 DM.

2 Almost the entire herd is infected, irrespective of calving number.

Date of inspection	L1 cows	Affected L1 cows	L2 cows	Affected L2 cows	L3 cows	Affected L3 cows	≥ L4 cows	Affected ≥ L4 cows	% L1 cows	% L2 cows	% L3 cows	% ≥ L4 cows	% affected L1 cows	% affected L2 cows	% affected L3 cows	% affected ≥ L4 cows
28/11/11	18	0	17	0	7	0	13	1	32.73 %	30.91 %	12.73 %	23.64 %	0 %	0 %	0 %	100 %
28/12/11	19	1	16	0	4	0	11	1	38 %	32 %	8 %	22 %	50 %	0 %	0 %	50 %
25/01/12	19	2	16	0	5	0	12	2	36.54 %	30.77 %	9.62 %	23.08 %	50 %	0 %	0 %	50 %
27/02/12	20	2	15	0	6	0	15	3	35.71 %	26.79 %	10.71 %	26.79 %	40 %	0 %	0 %	60 %
27/03/12	21	1	15	0	6	0	15	3	36.84 %	26.32 %	10.53 %	26.32 %	25 %	0 %	0 %	75 %
26/04/12	21	0	16	0	8	0	9	0	38.89 %	29.63 %	14.81 %	16.67 %	0 %	0 %	0 %	0 %
25/05/12	20	1	13	0	8	1	9	1	40 %	26 %	16 %	18 %	33.33 %	0 %	33.33 %	33.33 %
25/06/12	19	0	12	0	8	2	9	0	39.58 %	25 %	16.67 %	18.75 %	0 %	0 %	100 %	0 %
25/07/12	21	1	12	0	11	2	10	2	38.89 %	22.22 %	20.37 %	18.52 %	20 %	0 %	40 %	40 %
2								Mean	37.46 %	27.74 %	13.27 %	21.53 %	24.26 %	0 %	19.26 %	45.37 %

DM: Days in milk L1: first lactation L2: second lactation L3: third lactation L4: fourth lactation

- Increased rate of chronic mastitis, i.e. there has been an increase in the number of cows that had cell counts of less than 200,000 cells /ml in one inspection and exhibit over 200,000 cells/ml in the subsequent inspection.
- A high number of cows present new infections at calving, i.e. cell counts of over 200,000 cells/ml in the first inspection after calving.

Evaluation of the farm

Hygiene and comfort

After evaluating the farm, the following conclusions are reached regarding hygiene and comfort:

- The cleanliness and hygiene of the udders and legs of lactating cows are satisfactory, but the hooves are dirty.
- The farm has yards with relatively clean, but the cleanliness of the aisle that borders the edges of the cubicles is lacking. The farm does not use an automatic cleaning system.
- Dry cows and prepartum heifers share a yard and a rest area. The animals are clean, but the outdoor yard could be improved in terms of space and hygiene (Fig. 1).
- The milking parlour is suitably clean and hygienic.
- The cubicles are of the appropriate dimensions to allow the cows to rest comfortably (Fig. 2). However, they are poorly constructed: the material used for the base of the bed is hard and the thickness of the bedding minimal (less than 10 cm).
- Sawdust and calcium carbonate (unspecified percentage) are used as bedding, both in fine powder form. Bedding is replaced once a week.
- The back of the cubicle contains clumps of bedding material mixed with fresh faeces (Fig. 3).

Milking machine

After evaluating the milking machine and parlour, the following conclusions were reached:

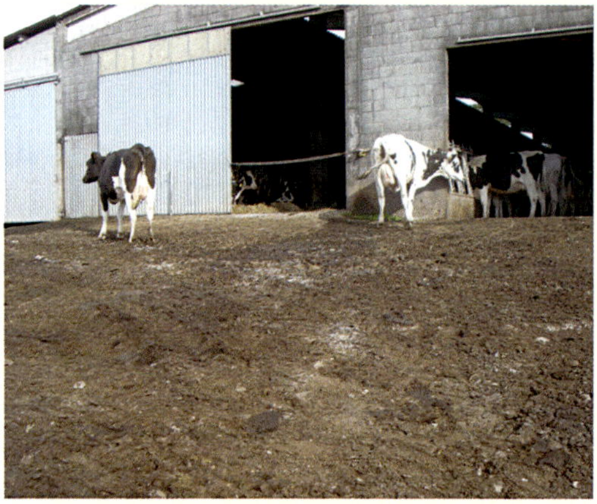

Figure 1. Dry cows and heifers share a yard and a rest area.

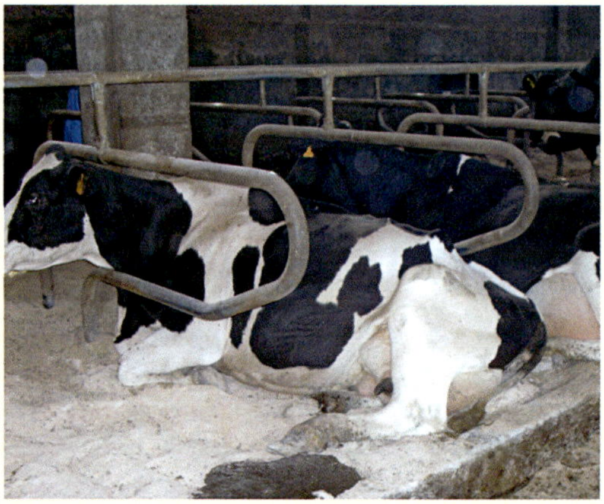

Figure 2. Good-sized but uncomfortable cubicle.

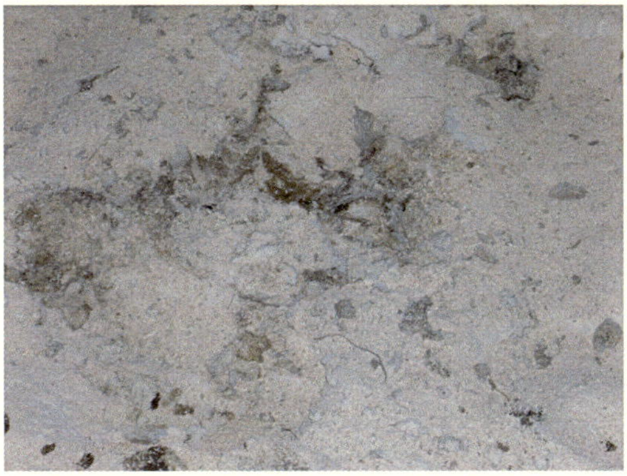

Figure 3. **Note the clumps of sawdust and fresh faeces in the beds.**

- The farm has a 5 x 5 herringbone milking parlour.
- The milking machine is a low pipeline, closed-loop design.
- The angle of the milk pipeline is inadequate and does not meet the required minimum of 2 % as stipulated in UNE 68061/98, which regulates the installation and use of milking machines.
- The alignment of the milking units during milking is incorrect. The cows are uncomfortable and kick.
- The teat cup liners of the milking machine are made of silicone and have seen 1,500 hours of milking.
- The milking machine creates a vacuum of 41 kilopascals (kPa). During milking, decreases of 5 kPa are detected in the manifold at maximum milk flow, which stabilises at 39 kPa at lower flow rates.
- Post-milking teat condition is good: no congestion is apparent, and the teat condition score is good (1.8), although 37 % of cows exhibit rings around the teat base after removal of the milking apparatus.

Milking routine

The milking procedure involves groups of five cows and is managed by two operators. The first operator discards the first jets of milk and performs the pre-milking disinfection (predipping). The second then dries the teats with a paper towel and the milking units are attached to each cow by the first operator.

After observing the farm's milking protocol, the following conclusions are reached:

- The predipping time is minimal: this process lasts less than 30 seconds.
- The product used in the predipping process contains no disinfectant.
- The duration of stimulation of the cow prior to teat cup attachment is adequate (90 seconds).
- The average milk flow rate is low: 2.8 L/min.
- The time between the connection of the first milking unit and the removal of the last is about 10 minutes.
- The cows' teats are well disinfected (sealed) after milking.

Analyses

Milk samples are collected for bacterial culture (Table 3) from cows with quarters that tested positive in the California Mastitis Test (CMT) and from those with clinical mastitis. Samples from the rest of the herd (Table 4) are taken for microbiological analyses (Table 5).

Samples of the bedding material are also collected. These include samples of stored sawdust/calcium carbonate as well as samples collected from the cubicles 12 hours after spreading (Fig. 4). The results of the bedding analyses are shown in Table 6.

Table 3. Results of bacteriological culture of milk samples taken from cows with CMT-positive quarters and/or clinical mastitis.

Microbiological analysis (sample per quarter)		
Cow	Quarter	Result
1	FR	No growth
2	BL	No growth
3	BL	*Klebsiella pneumoniae*
4	FR	*Klebsiella oxytoca*

FR: front right
BL: back left

Table 4. Results of bacterial cultures of milk samples taken from milking cows negative for mastitis.

Microbiological analysis (sample per cow)	
Cow	Result
1	CNS
2	No growth
3	CNS
4	No growth
5	*Enterococcus* spp.
6	CNS
7	CNS
8	CNS
9	No growth
10	No growth
11	*Enterococcus* spp.
12	CNS
13	*Klebsiella pneumoniae*
14	*Enterococcus* spp.
15	CNS
16	CNS
17	CNS
18	No growth
19	CNS
20	No growth
21	CNS
22	No growth
23	CNS
24	CNS
25	CNS
26	CNS
27	-
28	*Enterobacter* spp.
29	No growth
30	CNS
31	No growth
32	CNS
33	*Enterobacter* spp.
34	CNS
35	*Klebsiella oxytoca*
36	CNS
37	No growth
38	CNS
39	CNS
40	CNS
41	*Streptococcus uberis*
42	CNS
43	No growth

CNS: Coagulase-negative *Staphylococcus*

Diagnosis

In conclusion, the evaluation of this farm is based on several critical factors:

1. **The hygiene of the beds**

   The back third of the cubicles is dirty, and the bedding material highly contaminated.

2. **Batches of animals**

   Dry cows and prepartum heifers share the yard and the rest area. There is a hygiene problem due to dirty yards, which results in contamination of the cubicles.

3. **3. Milking machine**

   - The teat cup liners create a compression ring at the teat base after milking in 37 % of cases.
   - The pulsation ratio is 60:40 (milking phase/massage phase) and the milk flow rate is low (2.8 L/min).
   - The pipelines that carry milk from the milking units are too long, hindering proper alignment and positioning of the units during milking.
   - The time taken to remove the teat cup is too long.

Table 5. Results of bacterial cultures of samples taken from the farm's milk tank.

Microbiological analysis (tank sample)	
Microorganism	**Result (CFU/ml)**
Coliforms	0
Escherichia coli	20
Enterococcus spp.	20
CNS	350
Staphylococcus aureus	0
Streptococcus agalactiae	0
Streptococcus dysgalactiae	0
Streptococcus uberis	0

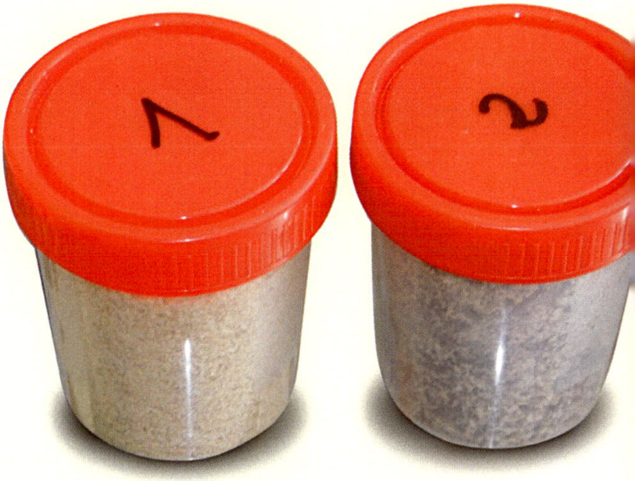

Figure 4. Samples of bedding material.

- The angle of the main milk pipeline is inadequate.
- The main milk pipeline of the system is too narrow.

4. **Facilities**
   - The beds are not sufficiently comfortable. The base of the bed is hard and the bedding thin (less than 10 cm). The waiting area has no ventilation or drinking troughs and does not provide the animals with sufficient space.
   - The exit from the milking parlour to the yard is inclined and slippery, and is uncomfortable for the cows, slowing their egress from the parlour.
   - The surface area of the drinking troughs in the lactation yard is not sufficient for the number of animals kept in the yard.

Table 6. Results of bacterial cultures of bedding samples.

Microbiological analysis (sawdust samples)		
Microorganism	**Result (CFU/g)**	
	Stored sawdust	**Sawdust from bed**
Coliforms	0	1,000,000,000
Escherichia coli	0	16,700
Enterococcus spp.	0	196,000
Total mesophiles	124,000	23,840,000
CNS	0	1,000,000,000
Staphylococcus aureus	0	0
Streptococcus spp.	0	1,000,000,000

CNS: Coagulase-negative Staphylococcus

5. **Milking routine**

A product with no disinfectant action (soap) is used when predipping teats before milking.

Recommendations

Short-term recommendations

1. Replace the bedding sawdust with another type of material. This is decided based on the presence of *Klebsiella* and other microorganisms in the sawdust. In this farm, it is not possible to use other inorganic bedding material (e.g. sand), as this would lead to problems in cleaning the aisles and draining manure into the manure pit. The sawdust is replaced with very fine calcium carbonate.
2. Thoroughly clean and change the bedding in the back third of each cubicle every day.
3. Provide a drinking trough in the milking yard and another in the milking parlour.
4. Change the teat cup liners, which have already reached the 1,500 hours of recommended milking use.
5. Reduce the time taken to remove the teat cups and change the pulsation ratio to 65/35 to improve the average milk flow rate.
6. Decrease the length of the milk pipeline and design a better system for the attachment and alignment of the milking units.
7. Use a hydrogen peroxide-based disinfectant for predipping.
8. Separate animals with clinical or subclinical mastitis and milk these animals last. If possible, these animals should also be separated in the milking yard.

Medium/long term recommendations

1. Improve the level of comfort of the beds by replacing the base material in the cubicles with a softer material, so that animals are more comfortable and do not slip when standing up.
2. Keep dry cows and prepartum heifers in separate yards.
3. Provide better ventilation in the waiting area.
4. Decrease the slope of the exit ramp from the milking parlour.
5. Increase both the angle and diameter of the main milk pipeline.

Treatments

The following drug treatments are recommended for cows with mastitis:

- **Parenteral antimicrobials:** 24 % solution containing trimethoprim (4 g/100 ml) and sulfadoxine (20 g/100 ml) at a dose of 1 ml/10 kg live weight.
- **Serotherapy:** hypertonic 7.5 % saline solution administered intravenously at 5 ml/kg live weight. Ensure that the animal is subsequently provided with drinking water.
- **NSAID:** flunixin meglumine (2.2 mg/kg of body weight).
- The **J5 vaccine** against *E. coli* is administered during the dry period and at the beginning of lactation.

Bibliography

Books

1. BENESCH, F. *Obstetricia y ginecología veterinarias*. Editorial Labor, S.A. Barcelona, España, 1965.

2. BLOOD, D.C., *et al. Medicina veterinaria*. Tratado de las enfermedades del ganado bovino, ovino, porcino, caprino y equino. Mcgraw-Hill Interamericana de España, S.L., 2001, vol. 1 y 2, 9ª edición.

3. BLOWEY, R.W. y WEAVER A.D. *Atlas a color de enfermedades y trastornos del ganado vacuno*. Elsevier España, S.A., Madrid, 2004, 2ª edición.

4. BURNELL, M., *et al. 21 Recomendaciones contra la metritis*. Pfizer Salud Animal, 2008.

5. BUXADE CARBO, C. *et al.* Bienestar animal y vacuno de leche*: mitos y realidades*. Ediciones Euroganadería, España, 2006, 1ª edición.

6. CORDERO DE CAMPILLO, M., *et al. Parasitología veterinaria*. Mcgraw-Hill Interamericana de España, S.L. Aravaca, Madrid, 1999.

7. DERIVAUX J. y EXTORS, F. *Fisiopatología de la gestación y obstetricia veterinaria*. Editorial Acribia, S.A., Zaragoza, España, 1984.

8. ELLI, M. *Manual Fatro de reproducción en ganado vacuno*. Servet Diseño y Comunicación S.L., Zaragoza, España, 2005, 1ª edición.

9. GARIJO TOLEDO, M., *et al. Atlas de patología parasitaria en rumiantes*. Merial Laboratorios S.A., 2012.

10. HOWARD, J.L. y SMITH, R. eds. *Current Veterinary Therapy*: Food Animal Practice, Philadelphia, PA: W. B. Saunders Company, 1999, 4ª edición.

11. QUINTELA ARIAS, L.A., *et al. Ecografía y reproducción de la vaca*. Servizo de publicacions e intercambio cientifico. Universidad de Santiago de Compostela, 2006.

12. ROSENBERGER, G. *Enfermedades de los bovinos*. Hemisferio Sur S.A. Buenos aires, Argentina, 1989, vol. I y II, 1ª edición (reimpresión).

13. SALAZAR, I. *Anatomía práctica del ganado vacuno*. Grass-Iatros Edicions, Barcelona, 1994.

14. VETESCAL. *Guía de orientación al diagnóstico ante problemas de calidad de leche*. Intervet/Schering-Plough, Madrid, 1ª edición, 2009.

Articles

1. BACH, A. y JUARISTI, J.L. Sistemas y prácticas de manejo en rebaños de vacuno lechero en España, XXIV Curso de especialización FEDNA, 2008, pp. 59-66.

2. Bouda, J., *et al.* Monitoreo, diagnóstico y prevención de trastornos metabólicos en vacas lecheras. *Bovinotecnia, Boletín técnico virtual,* noviembre 2005, p. 8.

3. Casamiglia, S. Nuevos avances en el manejo y alimentación de la vaca durante el preparto. XVI Curso de especialización FEDNA, 2000, pp. 45-66.

4. Dairy News. Publicación de Elanco Animal Health. Las etapas de la vida de la vaca lechera: objetivos, riesgos y recomendaciones. *Planeta Semex*, otoño 2000, pp. 6-7.

5. Dairy Cattle Reproduction Council. La monitorización de los niveles de NEFAs y BHB en las vacas en transición son un elemento clave para el control del balance energético. *Ceva Repro News*, abril 2012, artículo 1, p. 1.

6. González Garrido, A. Metabolismo hepático y vaca en transición. *Frisona española*, 2007, nº 160, pp. 116-119.

7. Jimeno Vinatea, V. El coste de la cetosis subclínica en la explotación de vacuno lechero. *PV Albéitar*, marzo 2013.

8. Linderoth, S. Impida que la metritis subclínica afecte a la mitad de sus vacas. *Dairy Herd*, abril 2008.

9. Meléndez, P. Manejo de la vaca lechera en el periodo de transición. Simposio Proyecta Bayer Chile, junio 2008.

10. Nydam, D., *et al.* Negative energy balance and Ketosis: Consequences and monitoring in transition cows. Department of Population Medicine and Diagnostic Sciences, Department of Animal Science, Cornell University.

11. Risco, C.A. Manejando la vaca posparto para maximizar la tasa de gestación. Universidad de Florida. *Planeta Semex*, otoño 2008, año 8, nº19, pp. 4-7.

12. Risco, C.A. Manifestaciones clínicas de las metritis posparto en vacas de leche. Secretaría de ANEMBE, agosto 2011.

13. Sales Nogueras, B. Manejo de la vaca seca. *Planeta Semex*, otoño 2009, nº 21, pp. 5-8

14. Sales Nogueras, B. Cómo gestionar la información en su explotación. *Planeta Semex*, otoño 2007, p. 1.

15. Santos, J. E. P. Pregnancy losses in lactating dairy cattle. *Rev. Med. Vet. Zoot.* 2009. 56:241-252.

16. Sirvén, M.H. Informe Técnico Nutrefeed. Manejo y alimentación de la vaca en transición.